A Colour Atlas of
OSTEOPOROSIS

A Colour Atlas of

OSTEOPOROSIS

John F. Aloia

MD, FACP

Winthrop-University Hospital
New York
USA

M Mosby

First published 1993 by Mosby–Year Book Europe Limited
Reprinted 1995 by Mosby, an imprint of Times Mirror International Publishers Limited
Reprinted by BPC Hazell Books, Aylesbury, England

ISBN 0 7234 1691 5

A CIP catalogue record for this book is available from the British Library.

Contents

Preface

Osteoporosis is a disease that is characterized by low bone mass (osteopenia) and micro-architectural deterioration of skeletal tissue leading to enhanced bone fragility and a consequent increase in risk of fracture. Although osteomalacia may have a greater world-wide prevalence, osteoporosis is a major health problem wherever longevity is a characteristic of the population. Thus, 75 million people in the United States, Europe and Japan are affected, including one in three postmenopausal women and most of the elderly of both sexes. The annual fracture rate due to osteoporosis is estimated at 1.3 million in the United States alone, with an annual health care cost in excess of 10 billion dollars. As the world population ages, the incidence of osteoporotic fractures will increase. The percentage of Americans older than 65 years by 2050 is estimated to be double that in 1981; it is expected that the incidence of hip fractures in that time will double.

The true impact of osteoporosis is appreciated by the finding that 6 months after a hip fracture only 25% of patients are fully recovered, whereas 50% need assistance with activities of daily living and 25% require long-term nursing care. The chronic pain and change in body image that accompany vertebral fractures and the fear of falling are also not reflected in any statistical presentation.

In the last decade there has been a knowledge explosion in the field of bone mineral research. Many forms of osteoporosis can now be prevented. Rehabilitative strategies, including effective medication, have been developed for the treatment of established osteoporosis. There is also reasonable hope that new medications which increase bone mass dramatically will be available in the next decade.

Acknowledgements

Louis, V. Avioli, M.D., *The Osteoporotic Syndrome: Detection, Prevention, and Treatment*, Grune and Stratton, Orlando, Florida.

Louis V. Avioli, M.D., *The Osteoporotic Syndrome: Detection, Prevention, and Treatment*, 2nd Edition. Grune and Stratton, Orlando, Florida.

Reginald Hall, BSc, M.D., FRCP, David Evered, BSc, M.D., FRCP, FIBiol, and Raymond Greene, MA, DM, FRCP. In: *Colour Atlas of Endocrinology*, Wolfe Medical Publications, England.

Reginald Hall, BSc, M.D, FRCP, David Evered, BSc, M.D., FRCP, FIBiol. In: *Colour Atlas of Endocrinology*, 2nd Edition. Wolfe Medical Publications, England.

Roger K. Khouri, M.D. Washington University School of Medicine, St. Louis, MO 63155. In: *JAMA — Tissue Transformation Into Bone In Vivo*, October 9, 1991. Vol. **266**, No 14, Fig. 1 and Fig. 2, pp. 1953–1955.

J. Joseph Melton, III, MD. Division of Endocrinology and Internal Medicine, Mayo Clinic, Rochester, MN 55905. *The Osteoporotic Syndrome: Detection, Prevention, and Treatment*, 2nd Edition, p.12, Figs. 1–3. Edited by Louis V. Avioli, M.D., Grune and Stratton, Orlando, Florida.

Victor Parsons, DM, FRCP. In: *Colour Atlas of Bone Disease,* Wolfe Medical Publications, England.

Robert Recker, MD. Metabolic Res. Unit, Creighton University, 601 N. 30th St., Suite 5740, Omaha, NE 68131.

Lawrence Riggs, M.D., Mayo Clinic and Foundation, 200, First Street, SW, Rochester, MN 55905. In: *The Osteoporotic Syndrome: Detection, Prevention, and Treatment,* p.12, Figs 1–3. 2nd Edition. Edited by Louis V. Avioli, MD., Grune and Stratton, Orlando, Florida.

Leon Sokoloff, MD. Pathology Department, State University of New York, Health Sciences Center, Stony Brook, NY.

Nelson B. Watts, M.D. The Emory Clinic, 1365, Clifton Rd. N.E. Atlanta, GA 3032. *Intermittent Cyclical Etidronate Treatment of Postmenopausal Osteoporosis,* NEJM, July 12, 1990. Vol. **323:**2, pp. 73–79, Fig. 3.

Colour Atlas of Metabolic Bone Disease, Mosby–Year Book Europe, Ltd., London, England.

Journal of Bone and Mineral Research Mary Ann Liebert, Inc. 1641 Third Avenue New York, NY In: *Journal of Bone and Mineral Research*, Vol. **7**:1, 1992, p.156, Fig. 2. Comparison of bone mineral content among Japanese, Koreans, and Taiwanese assessed by dual-photon absorptiometry.

Lunar Corporation, 313, West Beltline Highway, Madison, WI. *Bone Densitometry —Clinical Slide Presentation,* Slide 1–2.

Mayo Clin. Proc., **54**:701–707,1979. Reproduced with permission from Garraway W.M., Stauffer R.N., Kur!and, L.T., O'Fallon W.M.: *Limb Fractures in a Defined Population. I. Frequency and Distribution.*

National Dairy Council, 6300, North River Road, Rosemont, IL.

National Osteoporosis Foundation, 2100, M. Street, N.W., Suite 602 Washington, DC 20037 In: *Physician's Resource Manual of Osteoporosis*, p.7, Figs 8 and 9.

New England Journal of Medicine, 10 Shattuck Street, Boston, MA 02115-6094. **314**:1676–1684, 1986 with permission.

The American Journal of Clinical Nutrition, (Mary Ann Liebert, Inc.), 9650, Rockville Pike. Bethesda, MD. The Osteoporotic Syndrome: Detection, Prevention, and Treatment, 2nd Edition, p.79, Fig. 5-4. (AJCN **32**:540–549, 1979). Edited by Louis V. Avioli, MD. Grune and Stratton, Orlando, Florida.

The Journal of the American Medical Association, 535 N. Dearborn St., Chicago, Illinois 60610. Tissue transformation into bone in vivo, October 9, 1991 – Vol. 266, No 14, Figs 1 and 2, p.1953–1955

United States Department of Agriculture, Photography Division, Room 4404S, Office of Public Affairs,Washington, DC 20250-1300.

Thanks to:

Photography:
Joseph O'Leary
Joseph Carbone

Radiology:
Gerald A. Irwin, M.D.
Richard Losada, M.D.
Perry Mandel, M.D.

Pathology:
Virginia Donovan, M.D.

Garden City Hotel
Garden City, NY

Ken's Nautilus and Bodybuilding Center
285–261 Mineola Blvd,
Mineola, NY

Robert Sommerville,
Franwin Pharmacy,
127 Mineola Blvd.,
Mineola, NY

Janice O'Donnell,
Diane McGill,
Mary Gamble,
Nancy Bolte,
Margaret Marinelli,
Mary Sheehan, MD.
Linda Russo, M.D.

1. The biology of bone

The skeleton permits locomotion, protects internal organs, and serves as a mineral reservoir. Bone must be light to allow locomotion and solid to withstand fracture. Skeletal mass is influenced by demands for increased strength resulting from mechanical loading which is site specific, and for mineral homeostasis which is systemic and hormonally controlled.

The shape and mass of a skeletal region increase or decrease depending on the mechanical load placed on it. This adaptation process is called modelling. The process by which bone is continuously turned over is called remodelling. Skeletal mass may be thought of as being controlled by a mechanostat — a theoretical mechanism that controls bone mass to change upward or downward in response to mechanical usage. Provided there is a minimal effective stress stimulus there will be increased modelling and/or remodelling at the loaded site, resulting in an increase in local mass. However, the response to mechanical stress is modulated by hormones and is under genetic control, and it may also be influenced by drugs, toxins and diseases. Whereas mechanical loading is site specific, these latter modulators may affect the remodelling of the entire skeleton.

Bone is comprised of two types of tissue, cortical and cancellous (**1**). Cortical bone, which comprises 80% of skeletal tissue, is densely packed and surrounds trabecular or cancellous bone which consists of intermeshing thin body plates (trabeculae) that are in contact with the bone marrow. Despite its smaller area, cancellous bone has greater responsiveness to remodelling signals. There are also two bone surfaces — the external (periosteal) and internal (endosteal). Cortical bone is seen using different histological techniques: polarized light (**2**); microradiographs (**3**); and Bodian stain (**4**).

1

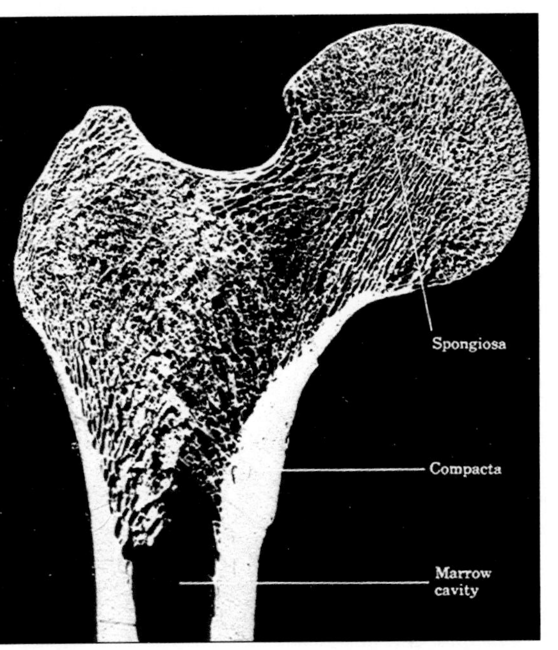

1 The two types of bone tissue: cortical and cancellous.

2

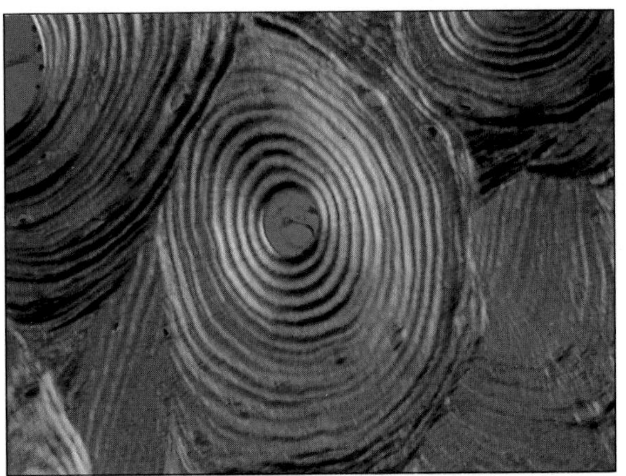

2 Cortical bone seen under polarized light.

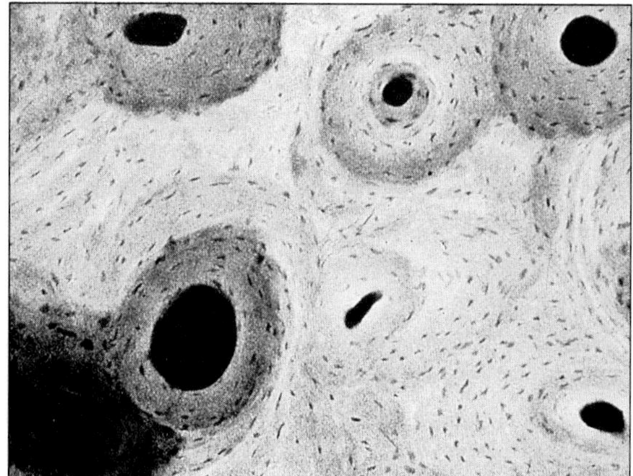

3 Cortical bone seen in a microradiograph.

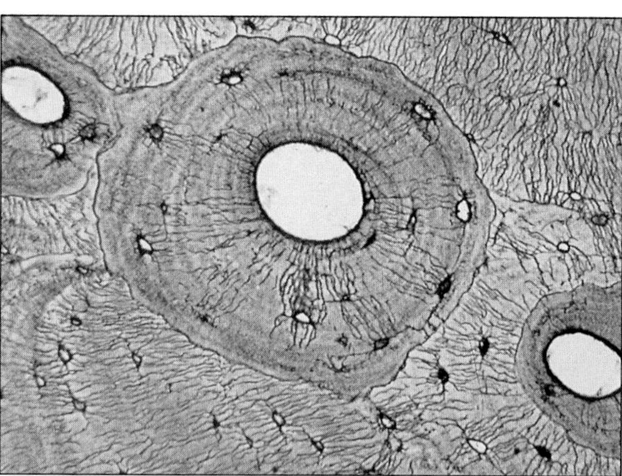

4 Cortical bone seen using Bodian stain.

The long bones have a greater proportion of cortical bone than do the vertebrae. Osteoporotic fractures in long bones tend to be in the areas where they have the greatest proportion of cancellous bone (the proximal femur and distal radius). The structure of bone is an orderly arrangement of matrix (collagen and ground substance) and mineral. Collagen fibrils overlap with the resulting spaces filled with hydroxyapatite (calcium, phosphorus, water). The alternating orientation of collagen fibres in layers gives bone its lamellar structure. The lamellae may be parallel to each other when deposited on a flat surface or concentric if deposited on the inner surface of a channel centred on a blood vessel (Haversian system). A central canal with blood vessels is shown in (**5**). When bone is formed very rapidly, as in Paget's disease, there is no preferential organization of the collagen fibres and so woven bone is produced (**6, 7**).

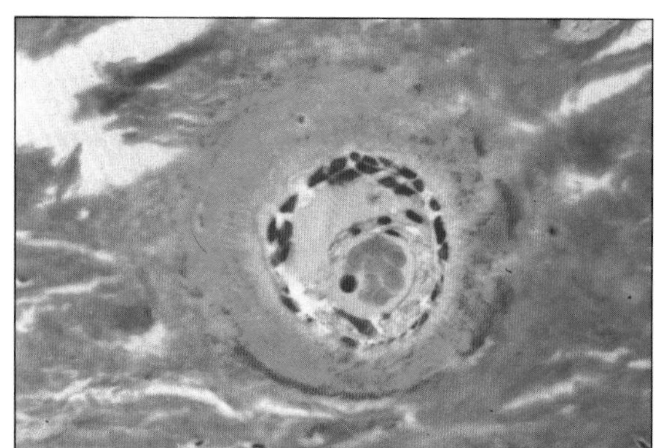

5 Haversian system showing a central canal with blood vessels.

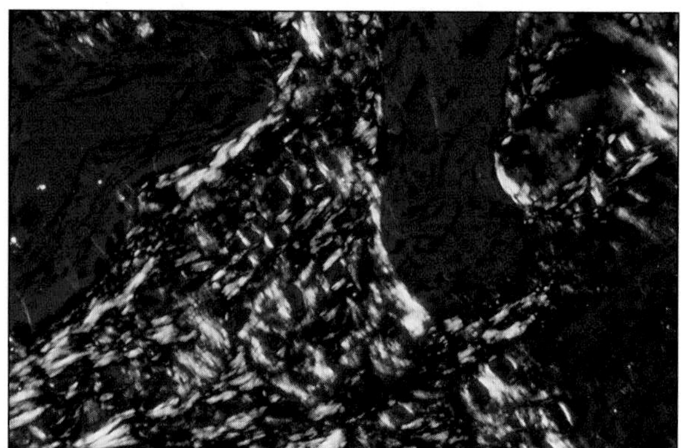

6 Woven bone seen under polarized light.

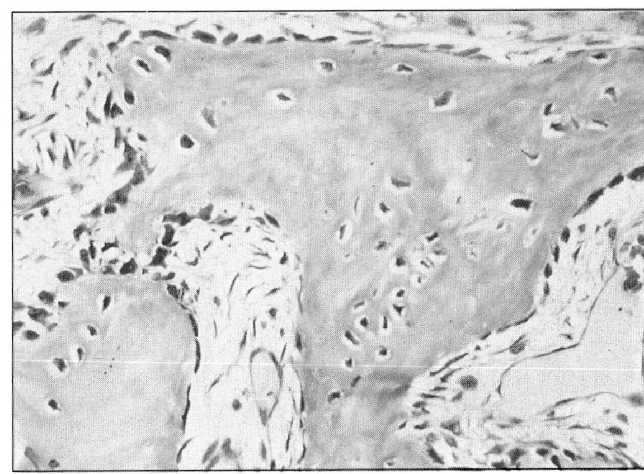

7 Woven bone.

When new bone is formed, matrix is deposited first and then mineralization occurs. The strength of bone is related to its mass and quality (matrix and architecture). Despite the presence of a normal mass, osteomalacic bone (with an increased amount of unmineralized matrix or osteoid) (**8–10**) may be less able to withstand mechanical loads, as is the case of osteosclerotic and fluoridic bone (**11**). In these instances there may be a normal or even an increased bone mass.

8

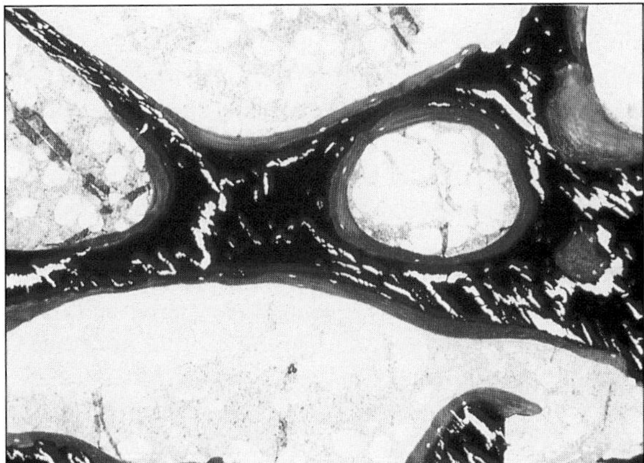

8 Osteomalacic bone shown using von Kossa stain.

9

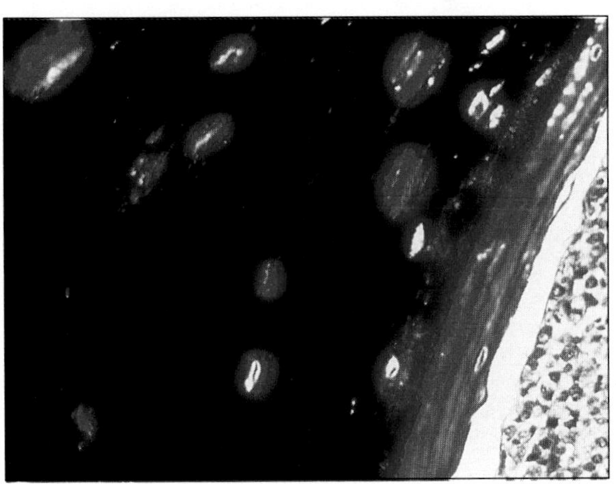

9 High-powered view of osteomalacic bone shown using von Kossa stain.

10

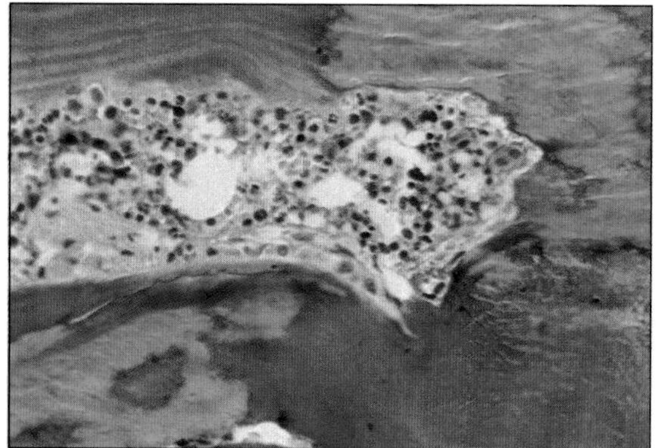

10 Goldner's stain showing the unmineralized osteoid as orange.

11

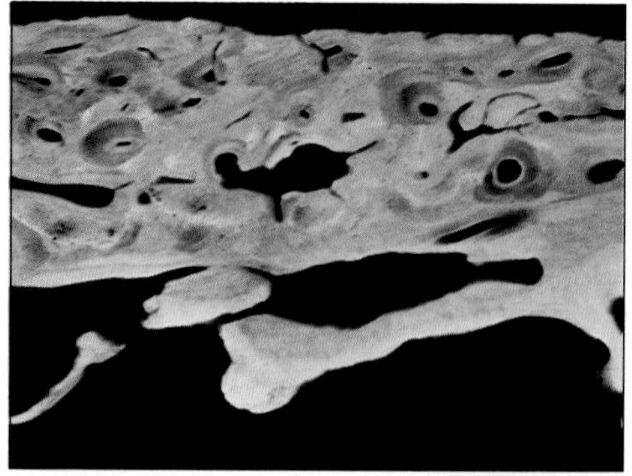

11 Fluoridic bone: despite increased mass, the quality of bone may be poor.

Bone tissue and bone cells

Bone remodelling balance can be positive or negative, resulting in a net skeletal gain or loss. Each year, 10–30% of the adult skeleton is replaced by remodelling This fulfills two requirements: the replacement of microfractures (microscopic breaks from stress); and maintaining mineral balance. Remodelling occurs in different stages and at different skeletal sites. Each site is referred to as a *remodelling unit* (typically there are over a million remodelling units). Bone remodelling is carried out by bone cells, i.e. osteoblasts, osteoclasts and osteocytes. Osteocytes are derived from osteoblasts but osteoclasts and osteoblasts have a separate lineage. The osteoblast (**12**) arises from resident progenitor cells and responds to growth factors, cytokines, and hormones (e.g., the fibroblast growth factor, IGF-1, TGF-ß, prostaglandin E, interleukin-1, parathyroid hormone, oestradiol, and 1,25-dihydroxyvitamin D_3). It is believed that the hormonal effects (at least of parathyroid hormone and oestrogen) may be mediated by growth factors such as IGF-1. Osteoblasts produce the bone matrix and have high levels of alkaline phosphatase. They also initiate bone mineralization.

Osteoclasts are multinucleated cells that are formed by the fusion of mononuclear haematopoietic procurers. The secretion of proteolytic enzymes across the ruffled border of the osteoclast on the bone surface results in dissolution of the bone (bone resorption) and development of a resorption cavity (**13**). A marked increased osteoclastic resorption may occur in disorders such as osteitis fibrosa (**14**) or Paget's disease (**15–17**).

12

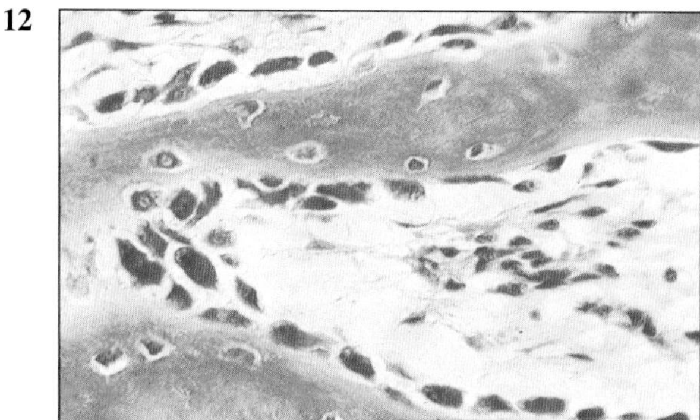

12 Osteoblasts lining the bone surface (*H&E* × 250).

13

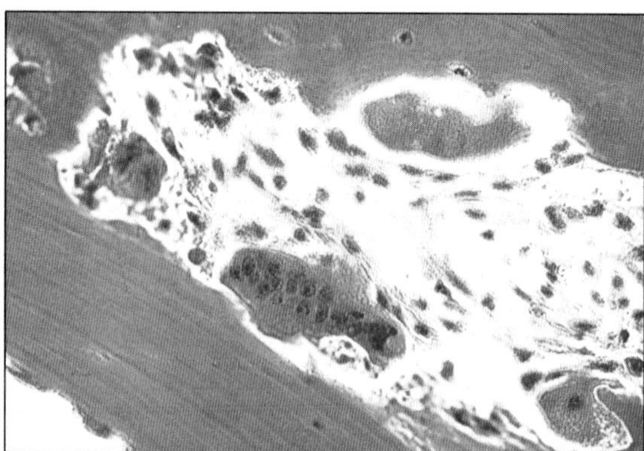

13 The development of a resorption cavity due to the secretion of proteolytic enzymes (*H&E* × 250).

14 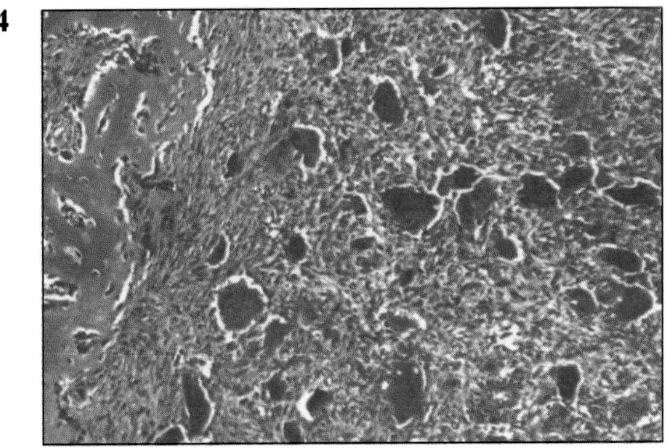

14 Osteoclastic resorption in osteitis fibrosa.

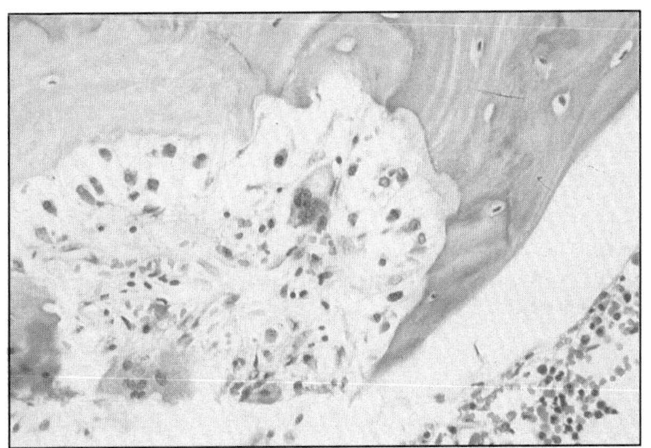 15

15 Osteoclastic resorption in Paget's disease.

16 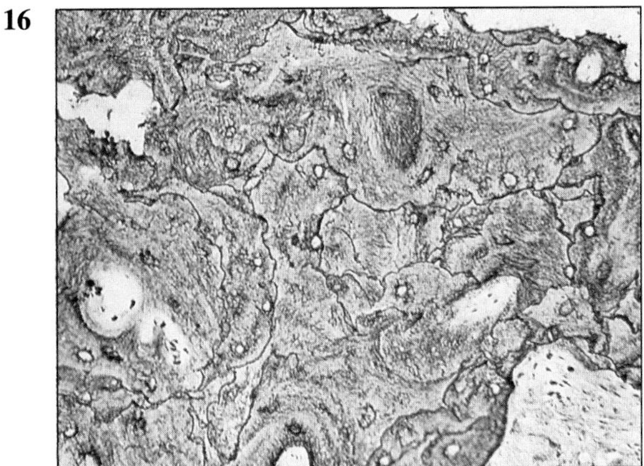

16 Paget's mosaic (Bodian).

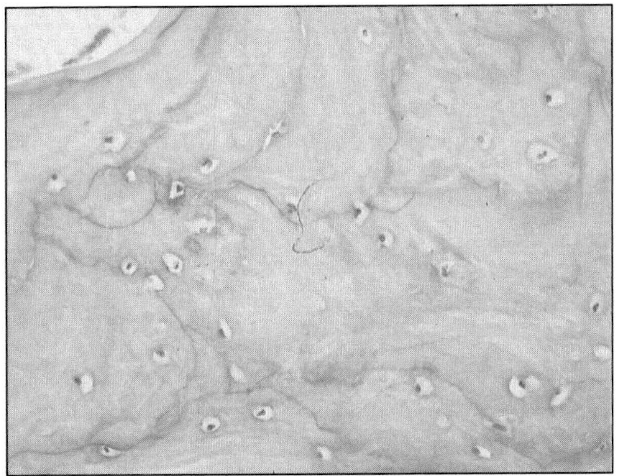 17

17 Paget's mosaic.

Some osteoblasts are internalized in the microcaniculi and become osteocytes (**18**). These develop cell processes that inter-react with each other and with the surface osteoblasts. It is believed that the osteocytes detect local mechanical loading and send signals to the surface osteoblasts to initiate bone remodelling. Osteoblasts have receptors for most hormones that influence remodelling except for calcitonin which has receptors on osteoclasts.

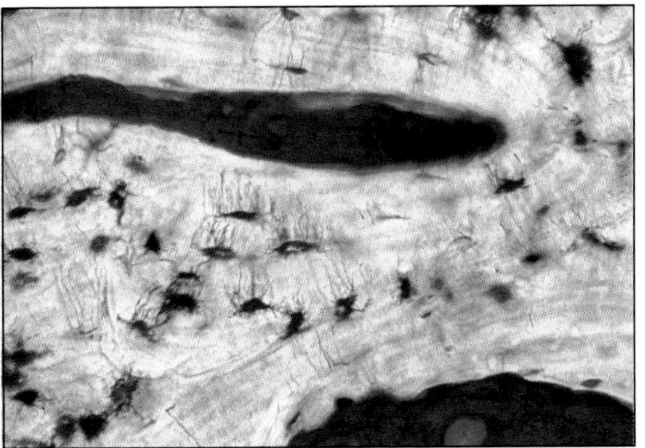 18

18 Osteocytes (basic fuchsin × 300).

The calciotrophic hormones

Circulating ionized calcium is maintained in a narrow range that is optimal for cell function. The maintenance of mineral homeostasis takes precedence over mechanical stimuli for the maintenance of skeletal mass. Parathyroid hormone has a negative feedback relationship with circulating ionizable calcium. Parathyroid hormone increases calcium absorption through the synthesis of calcitriol, the active metabolite of vitamin D; it increases bone resorption, and decreases urinary calcium excretion. Although the physiologic significance of calcitonin in man remains speculative, it protects against hypercalcaemic stimuli primarily by decreasing bone resorption. Other hormonal regulators of bone remodelling include sex steroids, thyroid, glucocorticoids, insulin and growth hormone. Since cellular events occur in discrete regions of bone it is likely that many effects of systemic hormones are modulated by local hormones; these are present in the micro-environment of bone and also have autocrine and paracrine functions. They include interleukin-1, lymphotoxin, tumour necrosis factor, gamma interferons, and transforming growth factors. Prostaglandins and bone morphogenetic factors may also play important roles *(Table 1).*

Table 1. Systemic and local regulators of bone remodelling.

Systemic	*Local factors*
Polypeptide hormones	Synthesized by bone cells
Parathyroid hormones (PTH)	Insulin-like growth factor (IGF-1)
Calcitonin (CT)	β_2-microglobulin (β_2-m)
Insulin	Transforming growth factor β (TGF-β)
Growth hormone	Fibroblast growth factors (FGF)
	Platelet-derived growth factor (PDGF)
Steroid hormones	
Calcitriol	Synthesized by bone-related tissue
Glucocorticoids	IGF-1 Basic FGF, TFG-β
Sex steroids	Interleukin-1 (IL-1)
	Tumour necrosis factor (TNF)
Thyroid hormone	
	Other factors
	Prostaglandins
	Binding proteins

The sequence of remodelling

The sequence of a bone remodelling cycle (which lasts from 100 days to 1 year or more) is shown in **19**. A signal (which can be mechanical or hormonal) is given to the osteoblasts which in turn give a signal to the osteoclasts to begin resorption over the next few days. Next, osteoblasts appear in the resorption cavity and deposit matrix, and then a mineralization phase follows *(Table 2).*

Table 2. Influences on activity of osteoblasts.

Increased activity	*Decreased activity*
Bone-derived growth factors	Glucocorticoids
Insulin-like growth factors	
Transforming growth factors	
Testosterone	
Prostaglandins	

19 Bone remodelling cycle.

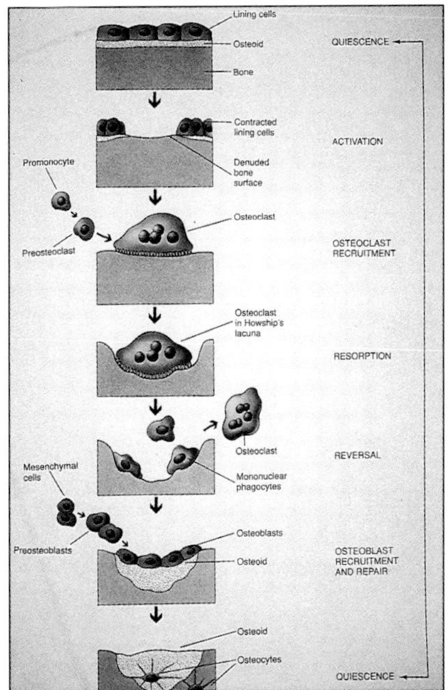

19

Bone formation continues for several months until the resorption cavity is filled. If the cavity is incompletely filled the remodelling balance is negative, and, if it is overfilled, it is positive. The depth of the resorption cavity may also vary and at times can transect an entire bone trabecula, resulting in permanent loss of architectural structure (**20, 21**). It should be appreciated that bone remodelling is a very complex activity and it has multiple feedback loops involving systemic hormones, morphogenetic proteins, local growth factors, cytokines and mechanical loading (*Table 3*).

Table 3. Activators and inhibitors of remodelling.

Activators	*Inhibitors*
Systemic	
Parathyroid hormone	Calcitonin
Growth hormone	Gonadal steroids
Calcitriol	
Prostaglandins	
Local	
Interleukin-1	Interferons
Lymphokines	

20

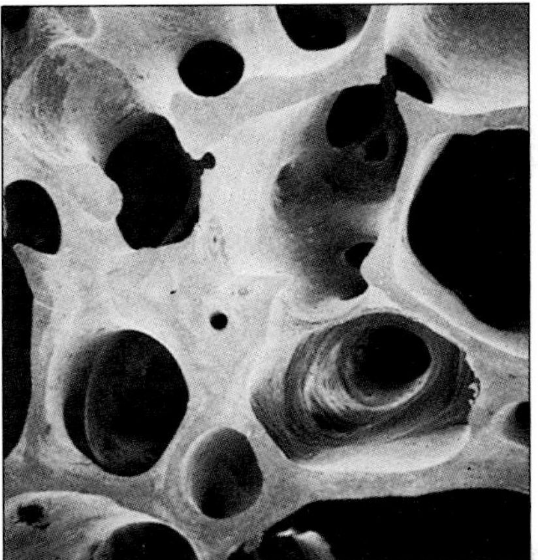

21

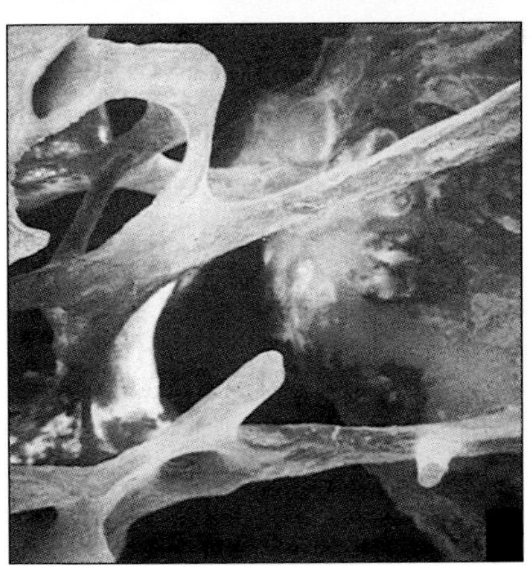

20, 21 Transection of bone trabecula.

2. Risk factors for osteoporosis and prophylaxis with hormonal therapy

Introduction

The reduction in bone mass in osteoporosis may be so marked that a fracture occurs simply from weight bearing. The reduction in the trabeculae of the spine is compared to a normal vertebra in **22**; vertebral collapse (loss of height) is seen in **23**.

22

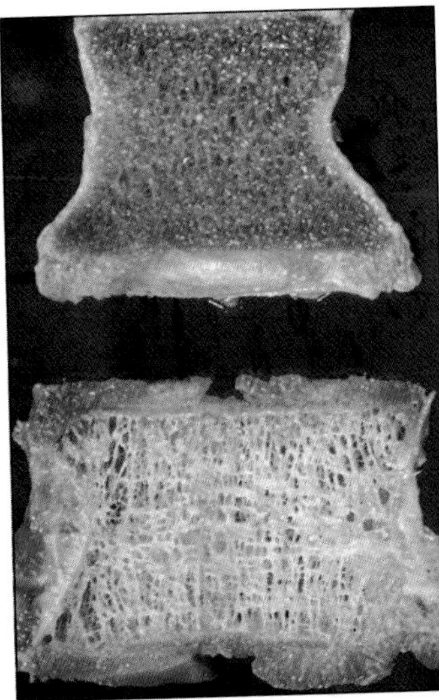

22 Comparison of reduced trabeculae of the spine with normal vertebra.

23

23 Vertebral collapse. Note the loss in height.

Although most hip fractures (**24**) result from falling, in some instances the patient's hip fractures spontaneously, causing the patient to fall. The loss of height from vertebral fractures is illustrated in **25** and **26**. The incidence of common osteoporotic fractures is shown in **27** and the percentage of cumulative incidence for men and women in **28**. The exponential rise in hip fractures with age in both men and women is apparent. From a prophylaxis viewpoint, it is important to realize that a delay in the rise of fracture incidence for just 5 years (through a manoeuvre such as hormone replacement therapy) will have a dramatic effect on the incidence of fractures in the elderly.

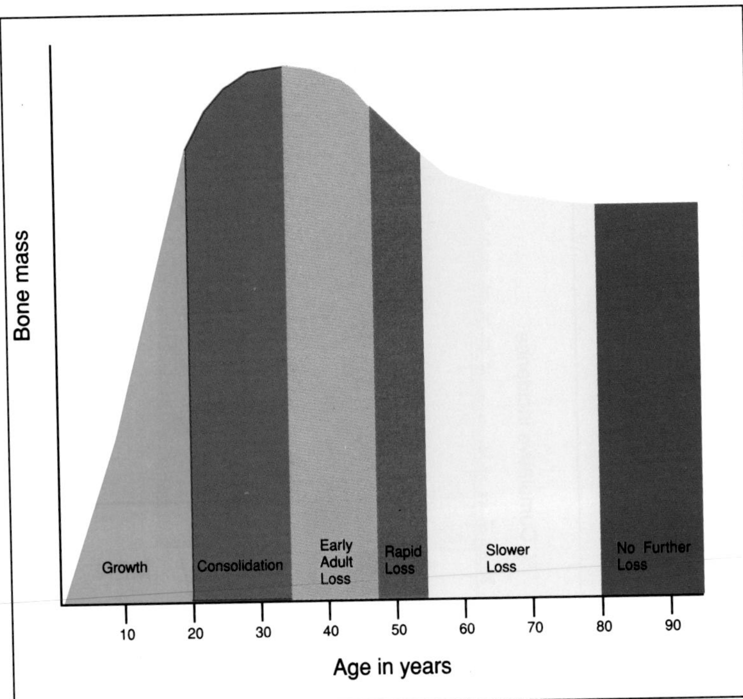

29 Graph illustrating phases of bone gain and bone loss during the life cycle. This graph reflects the total skeleton which is predominantly cortical bone.

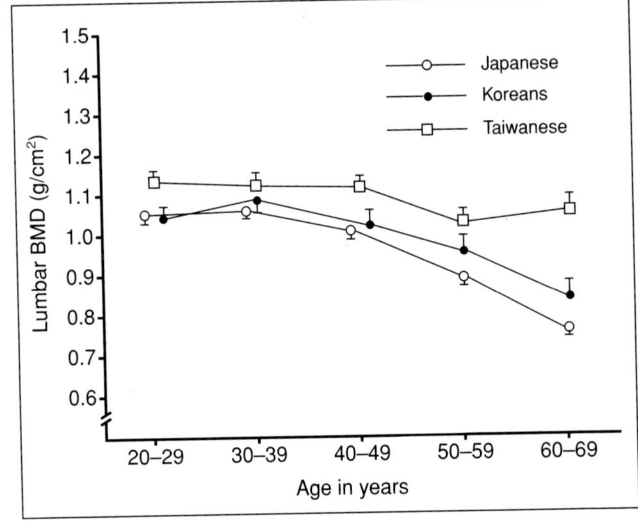

30 Graph comparing the bone mass within an ethnic group and showing different values in three different Asian countries.

The greatest increase in skeletal mass is during childhood. Under the influence of gonadal hormones, there is a rapid phase of skeletal growth during adolescence amounting to almost 45% of adult skeletal mass. There is evidence that, in women, the skeletal mass continues to increase until reproduction. This pattern of bone gain is primarily based on studies of cortical bone or of the whole skeleton which is comprised of 80% of cortical bone. Recent studies of cancellous vertebral bone density suggest that the difference between black and white girls occurs during puberty when the spine in a black girl shows a more marked increase in bone density than in a white girl. From birth to approximately 11 years old, boys and girls have the same bone mass, but by the onset of puberty girls actually exceed boys by 10–15%, with boys increasing during and after puberty. There is general agreement that maximal bone density is probably achieved within the second or third decade of life. These studies in adolescence emphasize the importance of gonadal hormones in all stages of the life cycle. Girls who exercise to the extent that they develop amenorrhoea, develop low bone mass. Spinal density is decreased even among women with regular menstrual cycles who have ovulatory cycles with changes in the length of the luteal phase. Boys with delayed puberty have osteopenia.

Attainment of the highest peak bone mass is limited by heredity. However, within this limit, maximal bone mass can be achieved by bone loading, an optimal calcium intake, and the avoidance of hypogonadism. In women, a slow bone loss seems to coincide with the decline in ovarian function; this may start gradually at an age as early as 30 years. There is rapid bone loss that continues for about 5 years after the menopause and which then reverts to a slower exponential rate, so that by the age of 70 years women again lose bone mass at the same slow rate as men. Whether this loss continues for life is controversial.

The loss of bone mass occurs at any time of the life cycle when oestrogen deficiency develops. Thus, women who have an oophorectomy at a younger age or premature menopause are at great risk of developing osteoporosis. Bone density is related to the length of time after the menopause (**31**). This oestrogen-dependent bone loss begins earlier in the spine and then in appendicular cortical bone. The change at the tissue levels from oestrogen deficiency appears to be an increase in the activation of the new remodelling sites with an increased activity of osteoclasts; this creates deeper resorption cavities which are incompletely filled with new bone by osteoblasts. The osteoclastic activity eventually perforates trabecular plates and completely eliminates them, not only lowering the mass of bone but also changing its architecture. It is unlikely that this rapid bone loss in the immediate perimenopausal years can be overcome by calcium supplementation of the diet since the bone resorption provides abundant calcium to the circulation. Moderate physical exercise is also unlikely to bring about a decreased rate of bone loss as the mechanostat is set at a higher level by gonadal hormone deficiency. Indeed, bone density values are much more closely correlated with the length of time after the menopause than they are with actual age.

Although bone mass is normally distributed in a healthy population and the risk of fracture based on bone density is a continuum, a frequently used clinical concept is that of a fracture threshold. This concept refers to a value of bone density that is so low that an individual is at high risk of fracture.

31

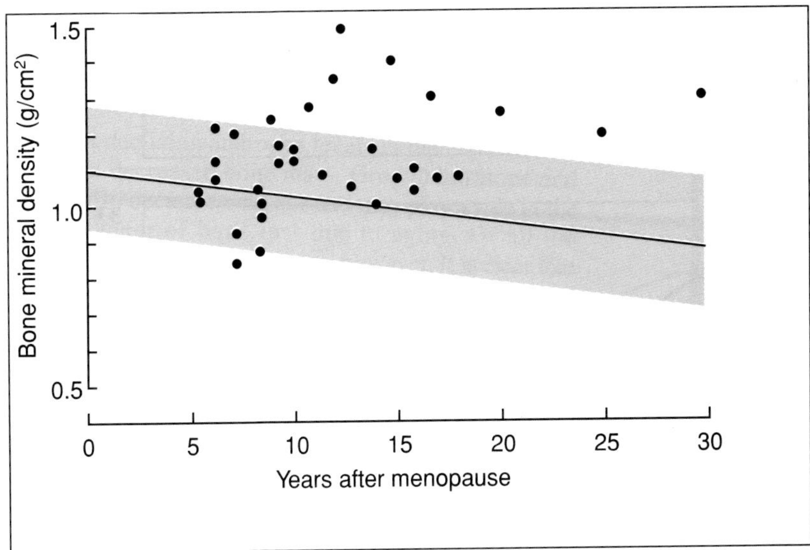

31 Graph showing the relationship between age after the menopause and bone mineral density.

Oestro

In recent y mass is ar later life. which hav bone mass

32

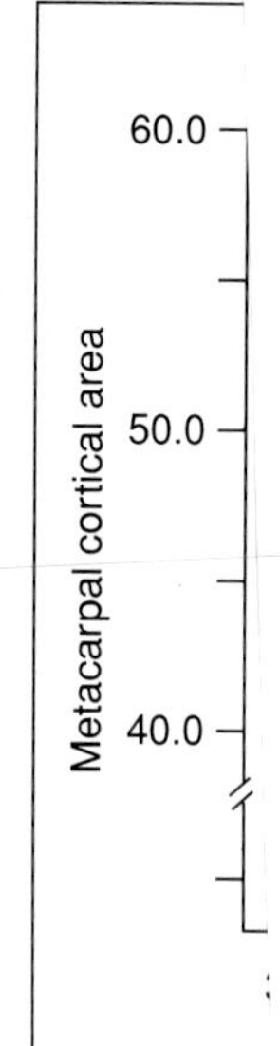

33

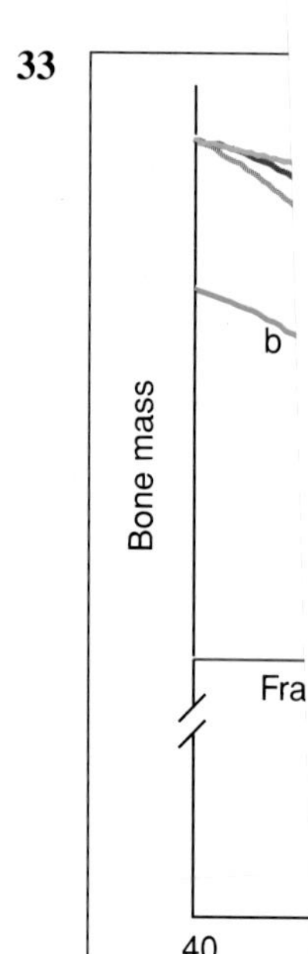

Bone strength

A bone density measurement can explain about 80% of the variance in bone strength. Other factors that are believed to influence the strength of bone with aging include:

- Reduced material strength.
- Inadequate microfracture repair.
- Altered bony architecture.

Perhaps the best example of a discrepancy between bone mass and bone strength is fluoridic bone which can have a markedly increased density and yet fracture more readily because of increased brittleness. Moreover, increased softness in patients with osteomalacia also predisposes to fracture. Microfracture repair is the repair of the fatigue or stress cracks that develop in most structural material and which also develop in bone. The number of microfractures increases with aging, particularly in areas of the spine subject to a great deal of mechanical loading (L2 through L4). Microfractures are repaired through bone remodelling. In women with postmenopausal osteoporosis, cross-bracing trabeculae are lost. However, in men all the trabeculae remain intact but become thinner. For an equal bone density this latter structure is stronger. The periosteal diameter of bone expands with age and the resilience of the shaft of the femur is reduced; the area that is most stressed is transferred to the proximal femur which is a common site for hip fractures. The loss of whole trabeculae of bone in cancellous bone also results in a disturbed bony architecture.

Exercise and bone mass

Bone loss occurs rapidly with the reduction of mechanical loading on the skeleton as is experienced by bed-rest or by space flight. Most cross-sectional studies and studies in athletes demonstrate a beneficial effect of physical activity on bone mass. These studies have led to the concept of the 'mechanostat' and suggest that skeletal mass adapts to the load placed upon it. This theory is similar to the negative feedback loops for control of hormonal secretion. Thus, bed-rest would result in less skeletal mass being needed to support the body. An increase in bone remodelling with increased resorption ensues, resulting in bone loss. Similarly, increasing the mechanical load results in a resetting of the mechanostat with increased bone formation. *In vitro* studies have shown the effects of exercise in stimulating osteoblastic activity via electromagnetic forces or through the increase or enhancement of cellular levels of growth factors. Cross-sectional studies of physical activity in premenopausal women have shown a higher bone density in those who are more active. In one prospective study of active, middle-aged women there was a 6.5% increase in spinal bone mineral density after 30 months training. Muscle mass has been shown to respond to exercise even in octogenarians. Prospective studies that have been done at various stages of the life cycle, however, have been equivocal in their results; some have shown an improvement of bone mass while others have indicated that exercise had no effect whatsoever. Although it appears likely that physical exercise is of value in promoting optimal bone density, there is insufficient information to prescribe an exercise programme to prevent bone loss with certainty. Moreover, with the withdrawal of exercise, bone loss will ensue so that the commitment to an exercise programme is a lifelong one. Although this may be undertaken by some individuals, the sedentary environment in developed countries and the high drop-out rate in supervised exercise programmes limit the utility of this modality of osteoporosis prevention.

Nutrition and bone mass

Calcium deficiency at any time in the life cycle results in reduced bone mass. The specific amount of calcium required during each phase has been a subject of great debate. The RDAs for calcium in the United States and Japan are listed in *Tables 4* and *5*. It is believed by many that these guidelines may be too low. One study showed that women with a high intake of dairy products have higher bone density (**35**) and a reduced likelihood of hip fractures (**36**) than women with a low intake. Several prospective studies have shown an interaction between calcium and other factors. They suggest that a lower dose of oestrogen can be used to prevent postmenopausal bone loss when dietary calcium intake is increased and that exercise increases bone mass only when calcium intake is adequate. Studies of calcium balance have shown that the average calcium intake associated with zero calcium balance was 500mg higher in postmenopausal women than in premenopausal women (**37**).

Table 4. Recommended dietary allowances, USA.

Category	*Age (years) or Condition*	*Vitamin D (μg)*	*Calcium (mg)*	*Phosphorus (mg)*	*Magnesium (mg)*	*Iron (mg)*	*Zinc (μg)*	*Iodine (mg)*	*Selenium (μg)*
Infants	0.0–0.5	7.5	400	300	40	6	5	49	10
	0.5–1.0	10	600	500	60	10	5	50	15
Children	1–3	10	800	800	80	10	10	70	20
	4–6	10	800	800	120	10	10	90	20
	7–10	10	800	800	170	10	10	120	30
Males	11–14	10	1,200	1,200	270	12	15	150	40
	15–18	10	1,200	1,200	400	12	15	150	50
	19–24	10	1,200	1,200	350	10	15	150	70
	25–50	5	800	800	350	10	15	150	70
	51+	5	800	800	350	10	15	150	70
Females	11–14	10	1,200	1,200	280	15	12	150	45
	15–18	10	1,200	1,200	300	15	12	150	50
	19–24	10	1,200	1,200	280	15	12	150	55
	25–50	5	800	800	280	15	12	150	55
	51+	5	800	800	280	10	12	150	55
Pregnant		10	1,200	1,200	320	30	15	175	65
Lactating	1st 6 months	10	1,200	1,200	355	15	19	200	75
	2nd 6 months	10	1,200	1,200	340	15	16	200	75

Table 5. Recommended dietary allowances, Japan (1989).

	Light activity						***Moderate activity***						***Heavy activity***					
	Energy (kcal)		*Ca*		*Vit. D (IU)*		*Energy (kcal)*		*Ca*		*Vit. D (IU)*		*Energy (kcal)*		*Ca*		*Vit. D (IU)*	
Age	*M*	*F*	*M*	*F*	*M*	*F*	*M*	*F*	*M*	*F*	*M*	*F*	*M*	*F*	*M*	*F*	*M*	*F*
15–19	2300–2400	2000–1850	0.8–0.6	0.6	50	100	2700–2600	2250–2050	0.8–0.7	0.7	50	100	3750–3700	3100–2850	0.8–0.7	0.6	50	100
20–39	2250–2200	1800–1750	0.6	0.6	50	100	2550–2500	2000	0.6	0.6	50	100	3550–3450	2800–2750	0.7	0.6	50	100
40–59	2150–2000	1700–1650	0.6	0.6	50	100	2400–2250	1950–1850	0.6	0.6	50	100	3350–3150	2700–2600	0.6	0.6	50	100
60–69	1850–1800	1550–1500	0.6	0.6	50	100	2100–2000	1750–1700	0.6	0.6	50	100	2850–2750	2400–2300	0.6	0.6	50	100
70–80+	1650–1500	1450–1250	0.6	0.6	50	100	1850–1650	1600–1400	0.6	0.6	50	100						

35

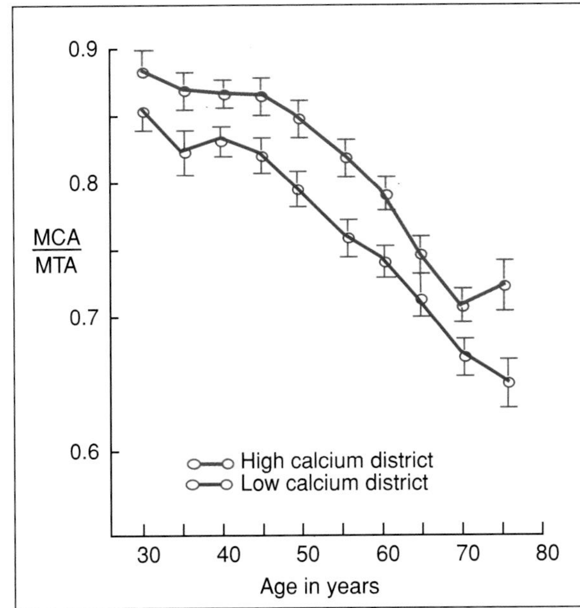

35 Graph comparing the bone density in women in two different regions in Yugoslavia. In the region where more dairy products are consumed the average bone density is seen to be higher.

36

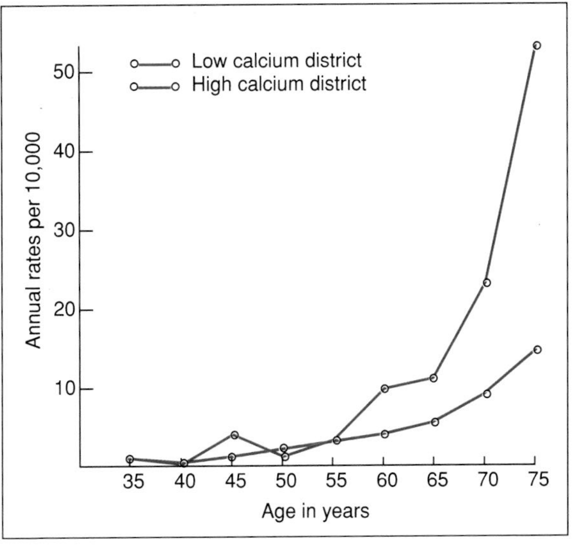

36 Graph comparing the number of hip fractures in the same groups of women as in **35** with the amount of dairy products consumed.

37

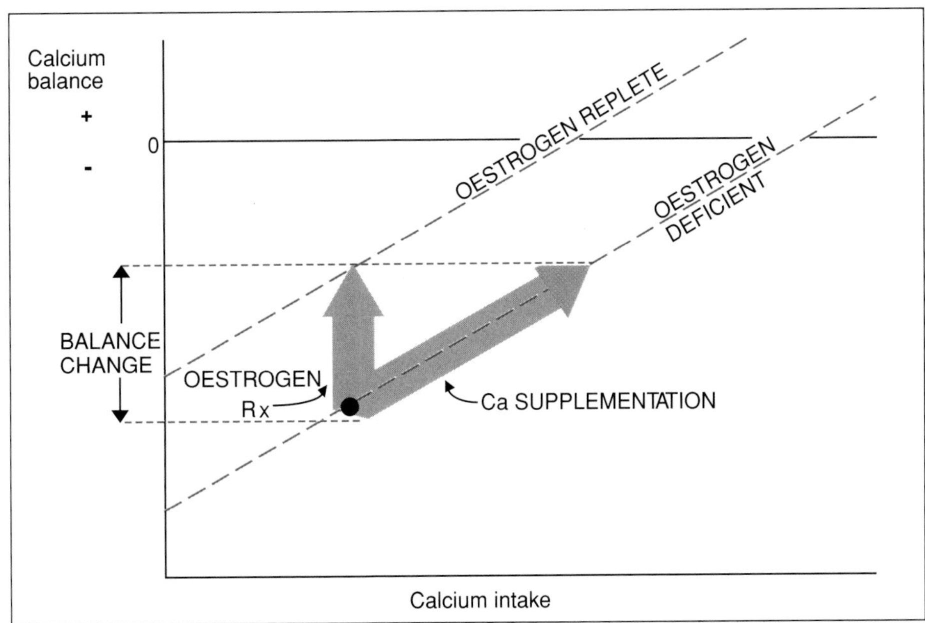

37 Graph showing the relationship between calcium intake, oestrogen status, and calcium balance.

Controlled studies suggest that there is a protective effect of higher calcium intakes in childhood and adulthood with the exception of the first few years around menopause. At menopause the oestrogen deficiency results in increased bone resorption, which leads to there being adequate calcium within the circulation; consequently, further bone loss is not prevented by providing more calcium. Indeed, clinical trials have demonstrated that calcium supplementation in the perimenopausal woman is ineffective when compared to oestrogen. Nonetheless, prospective studies have also shown that increasing calcium intake prevents bone loss in women 5 years after the menopause and well into later life. The benefit of dietary calcium supplementation was particularly noted in women who had a calcium intake of less than 400mg per day. The average intake in menopausal women in the United States is only about 500mg per day. In addition, in countries such as Japan where there is less bio-availability from the calcium-rich foods that are eaten, the intake may be even lower.

Adequate intake of vitamin D is also important in maintaining bone health. Deficiency of vitamin D, either nutritional or as a result of metabolic defects, results in rickets in children and osteomalacia in adults (**38, 39**). A mild deficiency of vitamin D may result in osteoporosis. Vitamin D intake is important in the elderly because their vitamin D dietary intake is reduced as is their exposure to sunlight. In addition, the renal ability to synthesise calcitriol is reduced with aging, together with the ability to absorb calcium from the diet. It has been recommended that supplements of 400 IU of vitamin D per day be provided to the elderly, particularly if they are housebound or have a low blood level of vitamin D. Elderly women lose spine bone density in the winter unless they receive this supplement. Frequent starvation diets will probably also lower bone mass. At the extreme levels, with an increasing number of adolescent girls with anorexia nervosa, this is readily demonstrable (**40**). High protein diets are also believed to increase urinary calcium loss but this has not been demonstrated as a factor in epidemiological studies. Excess dietary phosphorus may cause bone loss. However, the amount of dietary phosphorus required is much greater than that consumed by most individuals.

38

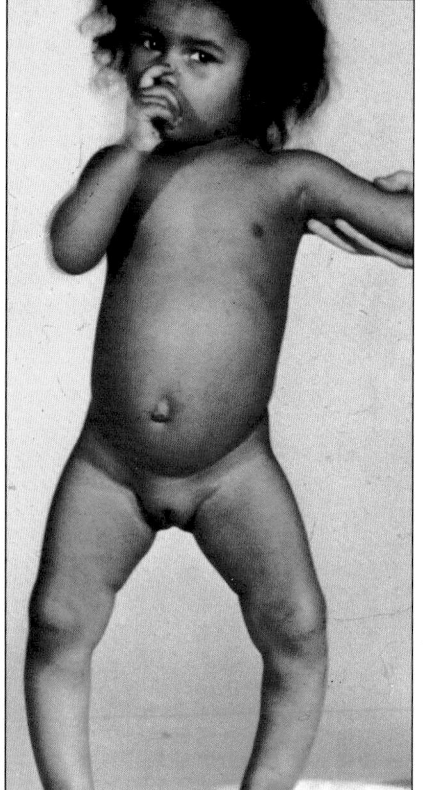

38 Rickets in a young child due to a vitamin D deficiency.

39

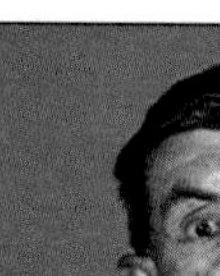

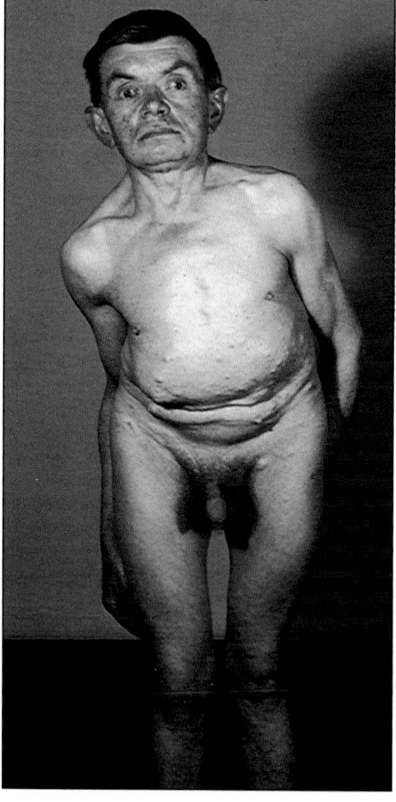

39 Osteomalacia in an adult due to a vitamin D deficiency.

40

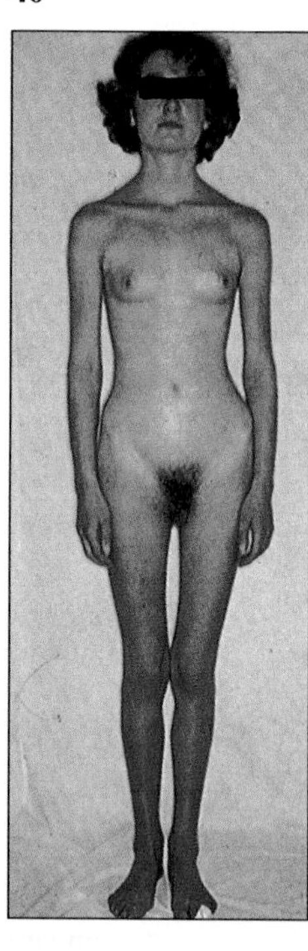

40 Anorexia nervosa is associated with bone loss.

The evidence linking bone loss to caffeine intake remains controversial; whereas excess alcohol on the other hand has been demonstrated to produce reduced bone mass and osteoporosis.

A fluoride intake of 1.5–4mg per day for adults is considered safe and may increase calcium retention and reduce the incidence of dental cavities. There is no convincing evidence that it is beneficial to exceed the RDAs for any of the trace metals. Excess sodium also increases loss of calcium in the urine. Sodium intake is higher in developed countries than is considered healthy for either the cardiovascular system or for bone. Because some types of fibre increase the speed at which the gastrointestinal tract empties there is concern that a very high fibre intake may decrease intestinal absorption of calcium. Fibre in recommended amounts probably does not have any effect on bone health. Oxalate and phytates are substances that decrease the bio-availability of calcium. Dark green, leafy vegetables, including chard, collards, spinach, beets and dandelion greens, have a high calcium content, but as a result of their oxalate content the calcium may be less bio-available. This has been definitively demonstrated for spinach. Other foods high in oxalates include asparagus, rhubarb, and chocolate. The Japanese diet, compared to Western diets, is higher in substances containing oxalate so that their dietary intake may result in lower bio-availability of ingested calcium. Phytates, because they are digested by bacteria in the intestine, probably do not have a significant effect on calcium absorption. Vitamins A and C, if taken in the range of the RDA, are sufficient for bone health. Individuals on strict 'vegan' diets, i.e. diets which eliminate all meats, fish, poultry, eggs, and dairy products, may be on a very calcium deficient diet. Clearly, individuals on such diets may require dietary calcium supplementation.

Cigarette smoking

Cigarette smoking has been clearly identified with osteopenia and osteoporotic fractures. Women who smoke increase their hip fracture risk by 1.7. About 10–20% of hip fractures are attributed to cigarette smoking. One mechanism whereby cigarette smoking contributes to osteoporosis is its effect on oestrogen metabolism. Women who take oestrogens have lower blood levels of oestradiol if they smoke. Moreover, women who smoke undergo an earlier menopause. Cigarette smoking is one of the factors why some women on hormonal replacement therapy continue to lose bone.

Drugs and illnesses

Many drugs are thought to produce bone loss. Glucocorticoids are some of the most obvious medications which produce a high frequency of osteoporosis. They have the following adverse effects:

- Reduce calcium absorption.
- Increase parathyroid hormone secretion.
- Increase bone resorption.
- Increase urinary calcium excretion.
- Decrease osteoblastic activity.

Hyperthyroidism produces bone loss as does thyrotoxicosis factitia. Since the development of the ultrasensitive assays for thyroid stimulating hormones (TSH) it has been shown that most people previously treated with thyroid replacement therapy were receiving excessive dosages. Some loop diuretics such as furosemide cause increased calcium excretion, but they are not clearly associated with osteoporosis. The prolonged use of aluminum containing antacids has been implicated in bone loss. Anticonvulsive medication interferes with vitamin D metabolism. Gonadatropin releasing hormone agonists used in the treatment of endometriosis also appear to produce bone loss.

Scoliosis is associated with osteoporosis (**41, 42**). The mechanism for this may be related to a genetic abnormality in collagen production. Any illness that results in poor nutrition or prolonged bed-rest can produce bone loss.

Other benefits of oestrogen treatment have long been established and include prevention of vulvo-genital atrophy and relief of vasomotor flushes and consequent sleep deprivation. The most important beneficial effect of oestrogen treatment is protection against heart disease. Oestrogen replacement therapy increases high density lipoprotein cholesterol, decreases low density lipoprotein cholesterol, and may have other beneficial effects on the coronary arteries. Analysis of the epidemiological evidence suggests that the use of oestrogen decreases the risk of coronary heart disease by about 45–50%. Absolute proof of this must await the completion of large scale clinical trials which are currently underway. If these clinical trials confirm this beneficial effect of oestrogen therapy, then the prevention of osteoporosis will be obscured as a benefit because oestrogen treatment will be recommended for all postmenopausal women who have no contra-indications for its use mainly because of the cardioprotective effect.

Progestogens have been used along with oestrogen and some progestogens have been shown to blunt the beneficial effect of oestrogen on HDL cholesterol. As a result there has been concern that the risk of heart attack may not, in fact, be reduced if progestogens are added. Initial studies, however, suggest that the combination of oestrogen and a progestogen does provide protection against coronary artery disease.

The risk of oestrogen therapy

The major concern with the use of oestrogen is the risk of developing cancer. One action of oestrogen is the increase in cellular levels of growth factors which may act as mitogens. It has been clearly shown that the use of unopposed oestrogen increases the risk of developing endometrial cancer by about two to five-fold. These cancers generally have a better prognosis than those arising in women not taking oestrogen. Indeed, these women have a lower overall mortality rate, possibly as a result of the lower risk of cardiovascular disease. When a progestogen is added to oestrogen replacement therapy there is no increased risk of endometrial cancer. However, cyclic regimens with oestrogen and progestogen often produce menstrual bleeding which is considered undesirable in many women and results in an increased need for uterine curettage with a higher rate of hysterectomy. As a result, there are some physicians who treat women with unopposed oestrogen and evaluate them periodically with endometrial biopsies; others use both continuous oestrogen and progestogens to prevent withdrawal bleeding and induce endometrial atrophy, thereby presumably preventing endometrial cancer.

The risk of breast cancer with oestrogen use is more controversial. A meta-analysis of epidemiological studies on the use of oestrogen for less than 10 years suggested that it did not increase the risk of breast cancer. However, studies of long-term use suggest a 30% increased risk of the diagnosis of breast cancer. It is believed by many that the more careful monitoring of women on oestrogen therapy results in earlier detection of breast cancer. In accordance with this view is the finding that women who develop breast cancer and who are taking oestrogen do not have an increased risk of dying as compared to non-users of oestrogen with breast cancer. The Nurses Health Study found the relative risk of breast cancer death was 1.1. Other studies have reported a lower risk of death from breast cancer among oestrogen users. Whether the addition of progestogens is beneficial in relation to the incidence of breast cancer is unknown.

Sophisticated analyses to evaluate the risk and benefits of oestrogen concentrate primarily on the accuracy of estimates of protection against coronary artery disease and of the increased risk for breast cancer. Other factors, such as the prevention of osteoporotic fractures and the development of gall bladder disease are of less significance. Prospective studies indicate that oestrogen users have a longer life expectancy than non-users. Unfortunately, for many women the fear of breast cancer will outweigh the benefit of greater longevity. At present the decision for hormonal replacement therapy can be made only with a well-informed patient taking into consideration her concerns, which may include the fear of disability from hip fracture, vertebral deformity or heart attack or the fear of development of cancer. A decision is aided in those who fear osteoporosis by performing a bone density measurement to determine the risk of future fractures.

All women started on hormonal replacement therapy should first have a mammogram to exclude the presence of an occult breast malignancy. For patients who have had a hysterectomy, a progestogen is not necessary. Hormonal replacement therapy should be continued for at least 5–10 years.

An oestrogen-dependent tumour is an absolute contra-indication to oestrogen therapy. Relative contra-indications include a recent endometrial malignancy, undiagnosed vaginal bleeding, active venous thrombo-embolism, and abnormal liver or renal function. Although fibrocystic breast disease is not a contra-indication, when fibrocystic changes are so dense that a small malignancy would not be detectable on mammo-graphy, or breast lesions have resulted in frequent biopsies, oestrogens are best avoided. Any dysplastic changes on breast biopsy or a history of breast cancer in first-degree relatives are reasonable relative contra-indications.

Prevention of injury

The probability that a bone will fracture is a function of the strength of the bone and the mechanical force applied to it (**46**). The majority of fractures in older adults are due to falls. Thus, the prevention of falls is important, as is the maintenance of an optimal bone mass. Only about 1% of falls result in a hip fracture in the elderly. The site fractured may depend on the direction of the fall (**47–49**). Japanese women have half the rate of hip fracture as whites in the United States, probably because they have been shown to fall on their side less often than white women. Whether a fall results in a fracture can depend on the neuromuscular protective responses that reduce the energy of the fall, and to local absorption of the impact by the fat and muscle surrounding the bone. Women with low risk for fractures have normal gait speed and normal arm extensor strength, whereas in elderly women gait speed is slow and arm strength declines so that they are more likely not to break the impact of a fall with an outstretched arm. Instead they are more likely to fall on their side and suffer a fracture of the femur. Thirty to thirty-five per cent of women over the age 75 years fall each year. Vertebral fractures can be influenced by the mechanical load placed upon the spine and the posture during weight bearing.

46

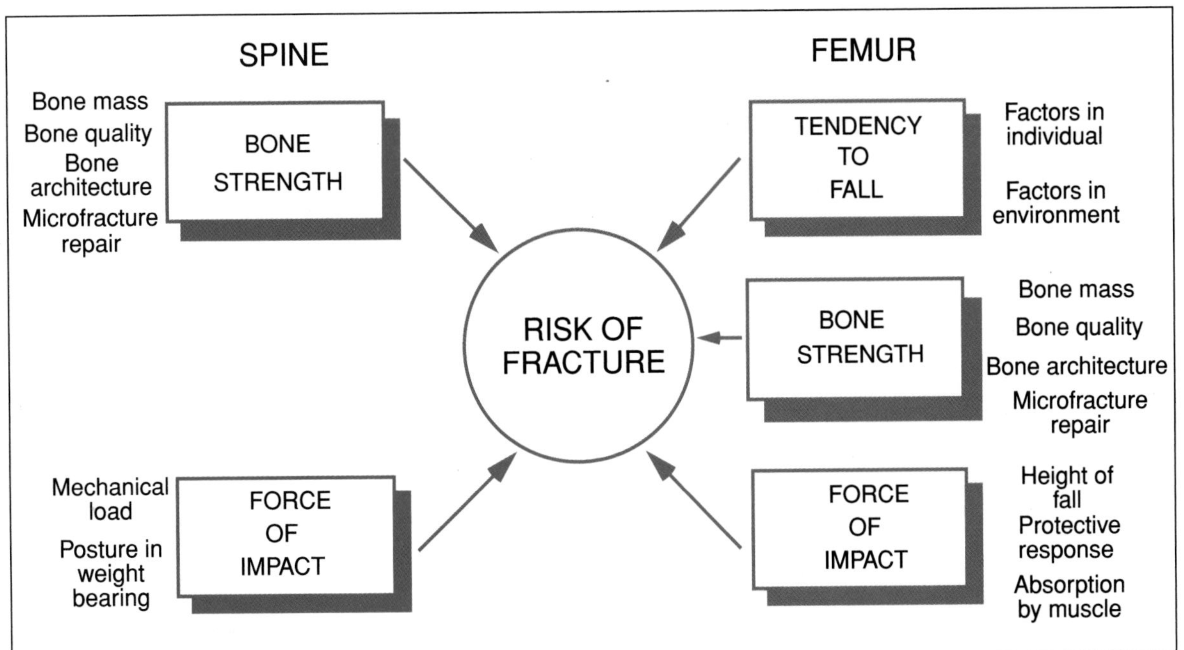

46 Diagram showing factors which affect the risk of fracture. The direction of fall is also a factor.

47

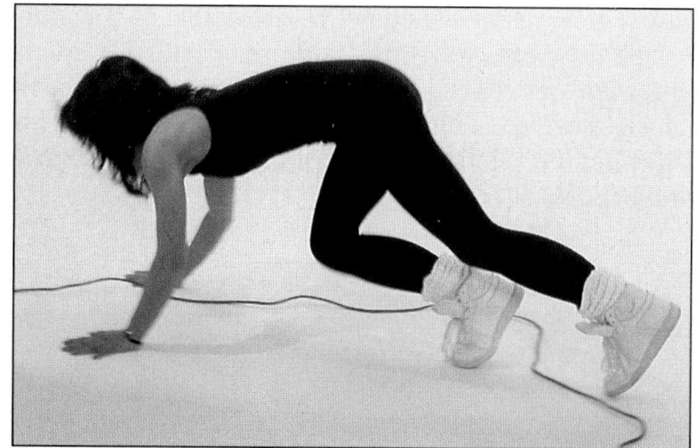

48

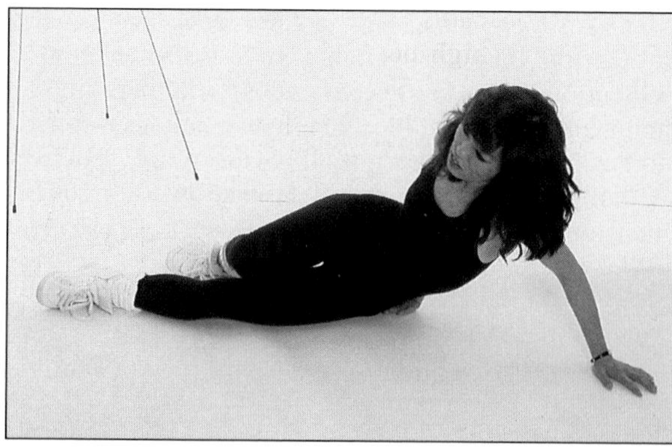

49

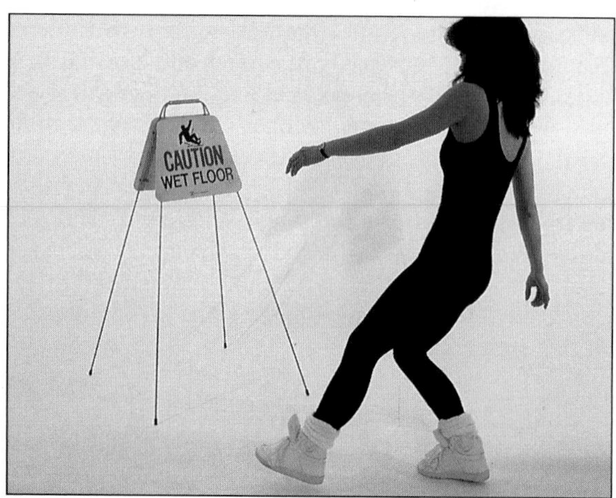

47, 48 Falling and using an arm as a support is likely to result in a Colles' fracture. A lateral fall can result in a hip fracture.

49 A fall backwards is likely to result in a spinal fracture.

The cause and prevention of falls

The causes of falls may be divided into intrinsic factors and environmental (extrinsic) factors *(Table 7)*. Intrinsic factors that make the elderly more prone to falling are : loss of postural control or increased sway; slow decision making; decreased alertness; decreased responsiveness; reduced peripheral perception; decreased vision; decreased hearing; postural hypotension; decreased muscle strength and tone; illness; arthritis; neurologic disability (including stroke and Parkinson's disease); cardiac arrhythmia; drop attacks; and vertigo. In addition, the use of long-acting sedatives and hypnotics has been associated with falls as has alcoholism. Extrinsic factors are associated with the environment, with the home remaining the most common site of fatal accidents in the elderly. Some factors include: slippery

Table 7. Factors increasing the propensity to fall.

Neurological	**Musculoskeletal**
Gait disturbance	Decreased muscle strength
Postural hypotension	Arthritic deformity
Vertigo	
Drop attacks	
Decreased alertness	**Cardiovascular**
Decreased awareness	Arrhythmia
Stroke, Parkinson's disease and cerebrovascular insufficiency	
	Drugs
	Alcohol
Senses	Sedative
Loss of vision	
Loss of hearing	

floors, slippery baths, lack of grab bars in the bath, low toilet seats, a high bed, inadequate lighting in the bedroom, loose rugs (**50**), and non-locking wheels on a bed. On the stairs, lack of handrails, poor lighting, high steps, and narrow stair treads can all be factors. In the dining room, inadequate lighting, slippery floors, and chairs with incorrect height with the lack of arm rests predispose to falling. Prevention of falls must include attention to both the intrinsic and extrinsic factors *(Table 8)*. Home safety is important. Examples of household safety tips are given in *Tables 9* and *10*. The use of a cane may improve stability in many elderly individuals.

Table 8. Fall prevention.

Obtain a fall history
Investigate medical causes of falls (cardiovascular, cerebrovascular, postural hypotension, muscoloskeletal)
Correct visual and hearing loss
Avoid alcohol and sedatives
Exercise for strength, flexibility and mechanical alignment
Dress warmly in cold weather
Wear low broad heels and non-skid footwear
Encourage the use of adaptive devices (cane, walking frame)
Avoid carrying heavy or awkward objects
Rise slowly—don't rush to the phone
Home safety rules

50

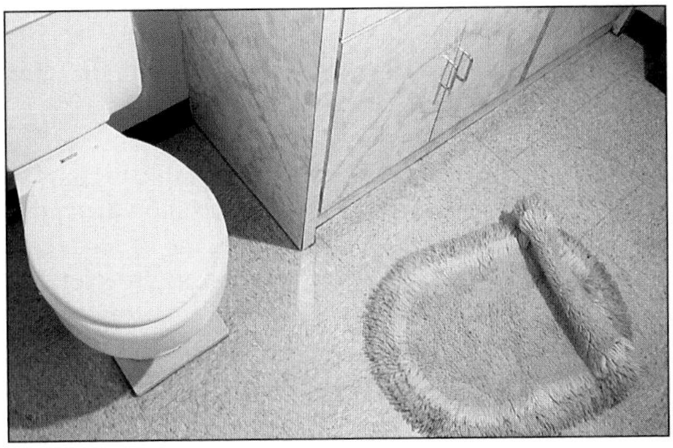

50 A loose rug could easily be the cause of a fall.

Table 9. Home safety: rooms in the home and outdoors.

Bathroom
Lighted pathway bed to bathroom
Raised toilet seat
Adequate water drainage to prevent slippery floors
Safety treads in bath
Kitchen
Have a sturdy step-stool
Use high chair for doing dishes
Telephone placed so that you do not have to run to answer
Living room
No throw rugs, frayed carpet or shag rugs
Seat height adequate for rising and sitting
Chairs stable, with arms
Do not use slippers or shoes with slippery soles
Bedroom
Bed low enough
No slippers or shoes with slippery soles
Have bedside tables for glasses rather than placing objects on floor beside bed
Outdoors
Avoid walking on ice
Avoid high curbs
Have walkways shovelled in winter and have salt and sand available for slippery surfaces
Use a cane if you are unsteady on your feet

Table 10. Home safety rules.

Lighting
Fluorescent or glazed bulbs in stairwells, bathroom, and night-light between bedroom and bathroom
Illuminated light switches outside each room
Walls, floors, stairs
Ensure sound handrails both sides of stair walls
Install handrails at front and back steps to house and near the bath, shower and toilet
Correct carpet irregularities
Keep objects off stairs and floors
Ensure sound stairs
Use waxless floor cleanser, avoid loose carpets, waxed linoleum, scattered toys, and pets
Clean spills quickly to avoid slipping

Avoiding injury to the spine

51

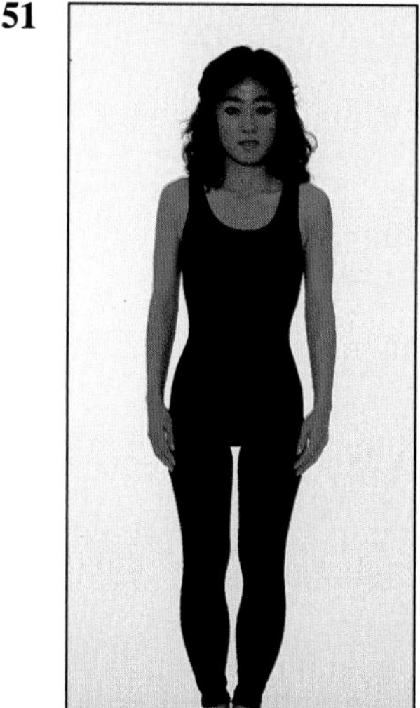

52

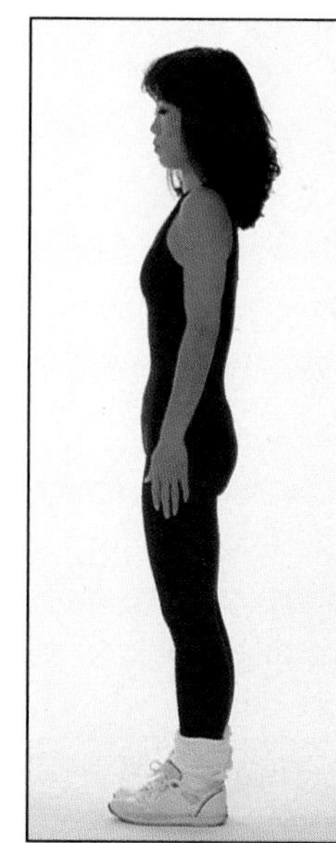

51, 52 The ideal standing posture.

The shape of the spine is arranged to minimize the effect of weight bearing. The maintenance of good posture (**51, 52**) protects the spine from fracture and also protects the intervertebral discs. The upper back should be flat whereas the lower back should arch backward. The shoulders should be back and pinched together toward each other. The head should be held high with the chin tucked in. Following a compression fracture of the spine, the natural curve of the spine changes so that there is kyphosis. This ensuing posture is undesirable because it does not properly distribute forces placed on the spine and results in more stress to the front of the vertebra and more likelihood of an anterior compression fracture. Flexion of the spine does the same thing. Therefore, for an osteoporotic patient to avoid vertebral fracture it is important to reduce kyphosis and increase lumbar lordosis, and to avoid spinal flexion and overloading the skeleton. Again, the home should be reassessed for potential areas where the spine may be injured. Automatic garage door openers should be installed, if possible. Window casings should be clean and lubricated. Pry bars should be used to loosen stuck windows. A reach should be used to pick up light objects. A pizza shovel may be used to move food around the kitchen. There are a variety of assistive devices that can be used to reduce or eliminate spinal flexion (**53, 54**).

53 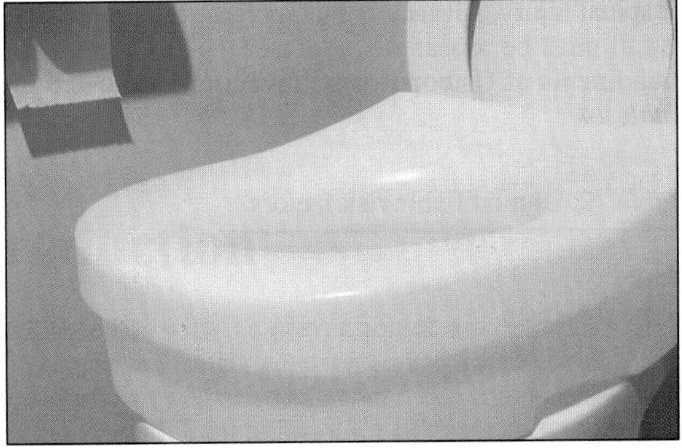

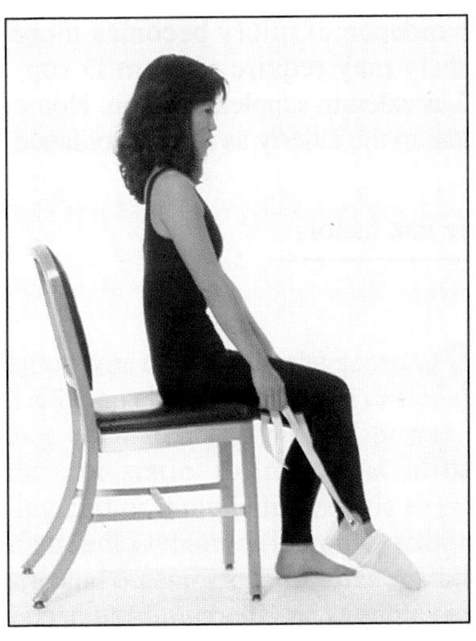 54

53, 54 A raised toilet seat and a sock valet are useful devices which reduce or eliminate spinal flexion. Others such as a 'reach' and long shoehorn also help.

Established risk factors for osteoporosis

Much of the evidence for a role of some of the factors described above in the pathogenesis of osteoporosis is inferential. Established risk factors for osteoporosis from epidemiological studies include: female sex, increasing age, Caucasian, oophorectomy at an early age, prolonged use of glucocorticoid steroids, and prolonged immobility. Gonadal insufficiency at any time of life is a risk factor as is a very low calcium diet (<400mg calcium per day). Cigarette smoking and alcoholism are risk factors. Protective effects are exercise, increased calcium intake, avoidance of obesity, hormonal replacement therapy, vitamin D intake, fluoride levels of 2 p.p.m. or more in drinking water, pregnancy, use of thiazide diuretics, and progestogens. These are the factors that, if modifiable, should be stressed in altering lifestyle habits in a preventive programme. An example of a woman at high risk of osteoporosis is illustrated in (**55**).In addition to good health habits, the major modifiable factors involve oestrogen, exercise and nutrition.

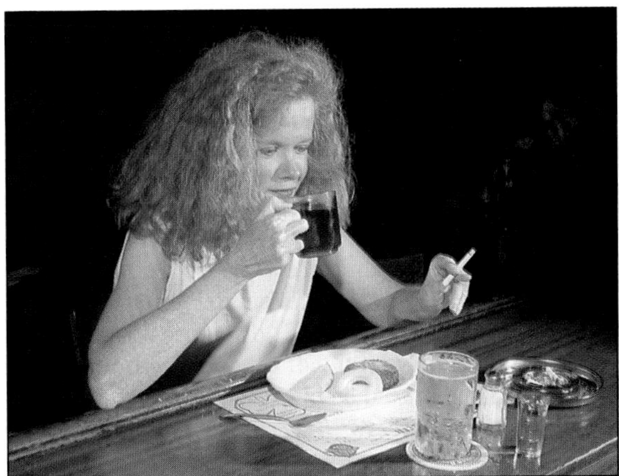 55

55 A woman at high risk of osteoporosis. She is fair skinned with small bones, does not exercise, drinks alcohol, smokes and ingests an unhealthy diet high in caffeine, salt and protein and low in calcium.

Strategy for lifelong prevention of osteoporotic fractures

Risk factors are modifiable and unmodifiable *(Tables 11* and *12)*. The modifiable risk factors for osteoporosis should be approached during each phase in the life cycle *(Table 13)*. Weight-bearing exercise, as well as exercise to improve co-ordination and flexibility is important at all stages of the life cycle. An adequate calcium intake is also important in all stages as is the avoidance of gonadal insufficiency. Promoting a healthy lifestyle, including the avoidance of tobacco and excess alcohol consumption, is the objective.

a cycle or stair step climber or rowing machine for 15 minutes daily, maintaining the target heart rate. Whatever exercise programme is prescribed, it must consider the patient's health, current fitness, body composition, and specific disabilities. Where appropriate, a stress electrocardiogram should be performed prior to initiating the programme. It is more likely that individuals will exercise successfully if:

- The exercise is supervised or in a group.
- Is indoors.
- Is made enjoyable.
- An exercise log is kept.
- The programme is increased slowly.
- The programme is demonstrated.

Exercise can eventually be continued using a home gym. It is important to recall that for a programme to work, other factors must be considered, e.g. exercise that produces amenorrhoea or is accompanied by a hypocaloric low calcium diet may result in bone loss. Daily exercise of at least one hour's duration is recommended. The following sections (*A–D*) give an example of an exercise programme for the prevention of osteoporosis.

A. *Warm-up and cool-down exercises*

Warm-up and cool-down exercises should last from 8–15 minutes. They should begin with stretching, postural, flexibility, calisthenics, and stress-reduction (such as T'ai Chi walk) exercises. Start with practising posture walking with a pillow on the head and follow with a T'ai Chi walk (**56–64**).

56

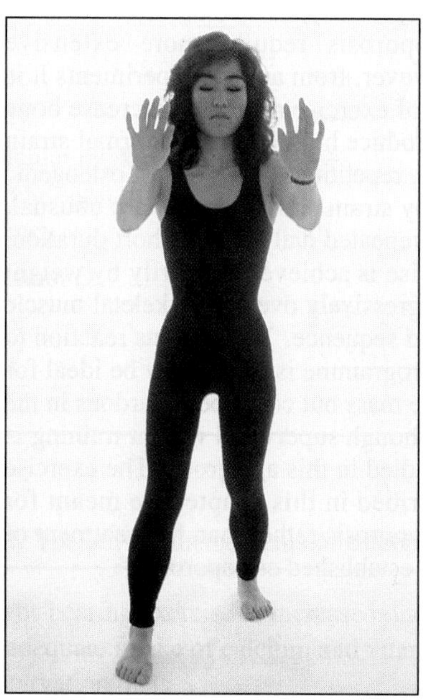

57

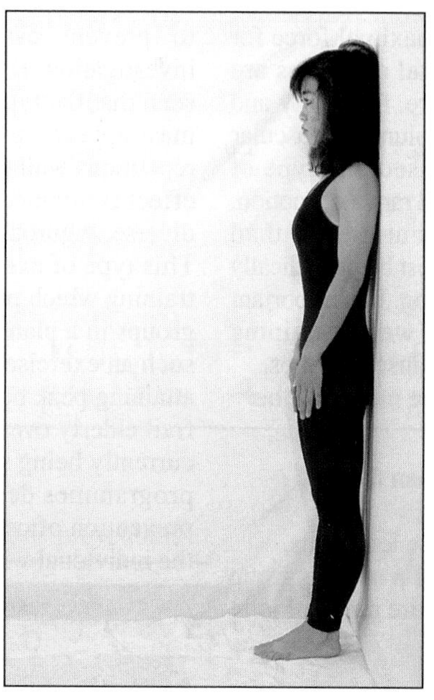

58

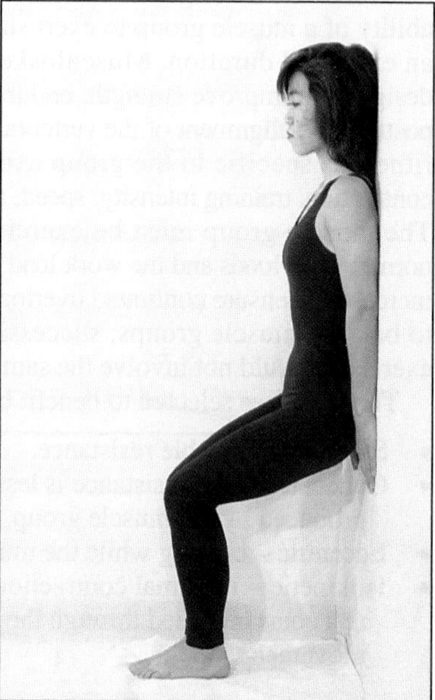

56 T'ai Chi walk. Feet straight forward, knees slightly bent and rotated outward over feet, stomach flat, chest forward and buttocks back, chin in. Breathe while gently raising arms, breathe out and return arms to starting position. Breathe in and raise arms as you slide heel forward, keeping back knee bent. Breathe out and push forward with arms as you step on to front foot, keeping body upright, not leaning forward. Breathe in and out slightly; lift arms as you draw the back foot forward. Breathe out as you place your foot flat and in line with the other foot, dropping your arms as you do so. Return to starting position. There are a variety of T'ai Chi exercises which may be done to increase flexibility and reduce stress.

57 Stand tall. Stand with the back against the wall; squeeze the shoulder blades together, tighten the abdominal muscles, place the lower back against the wall, and lift the head high. *Repeat 10 times.*

58 Wall glide. In the same position, bend your knees into a slightly squatting position and return to upright position. *Repeat 10 times.*

59

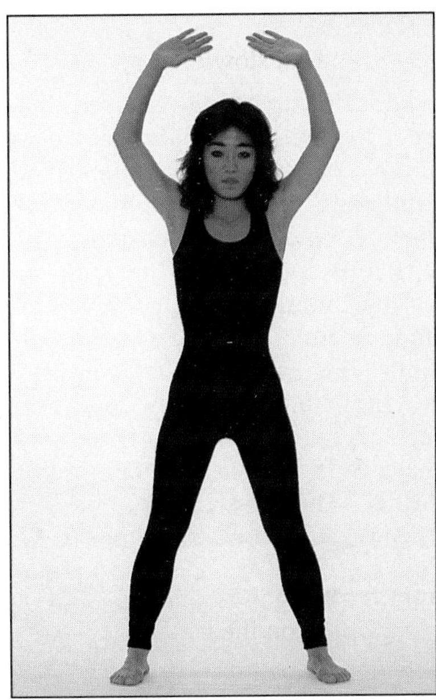

60

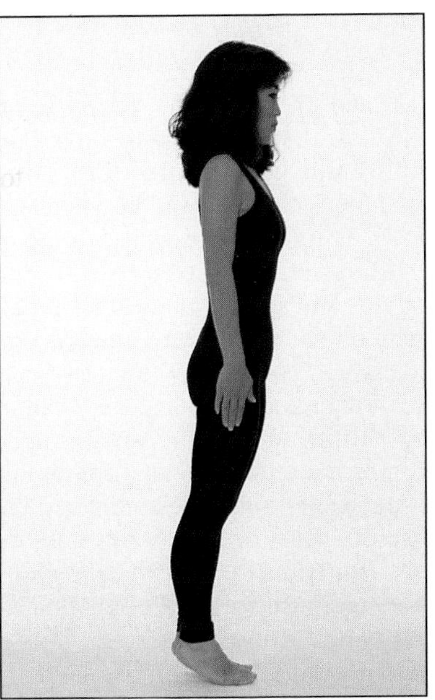

61

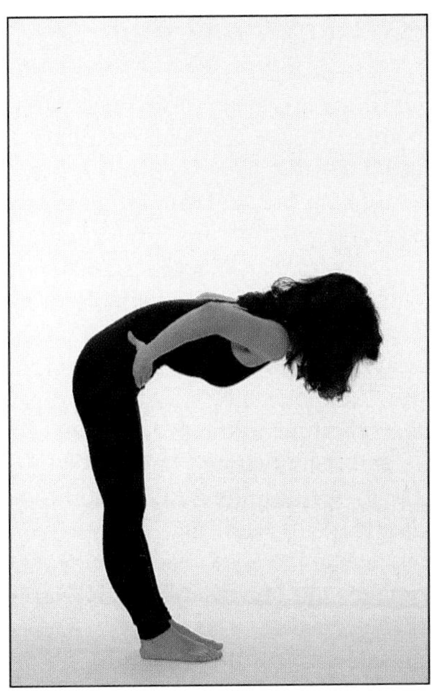

59 Jumping jacks. Swing the arms over the head and spread the feet apart in one movement. Then return to the starting position. *Repeat 20 times.*

60 Heel raises. With your feet apart, raise to a toe position, then lower your body. *Repeat 15 times.*

61 Forward bend. Stand astride with your hands on your hips and bend slowly to a 90° angle. Return slowly to an erect position. *Repeat 10 times.*

62

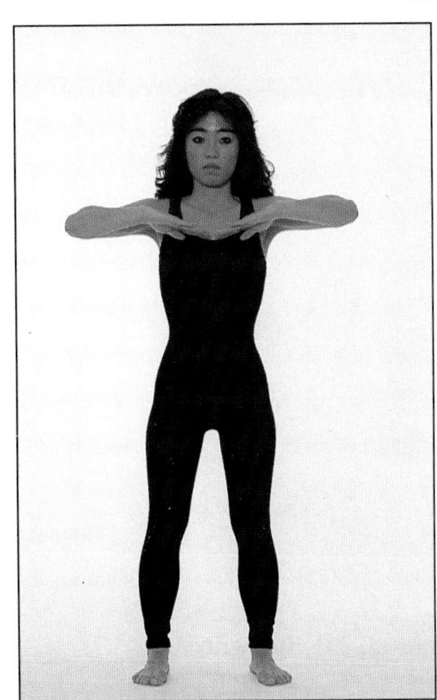

63

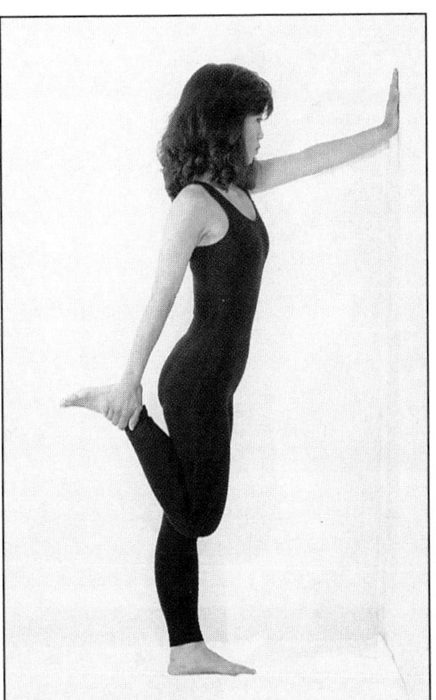

64

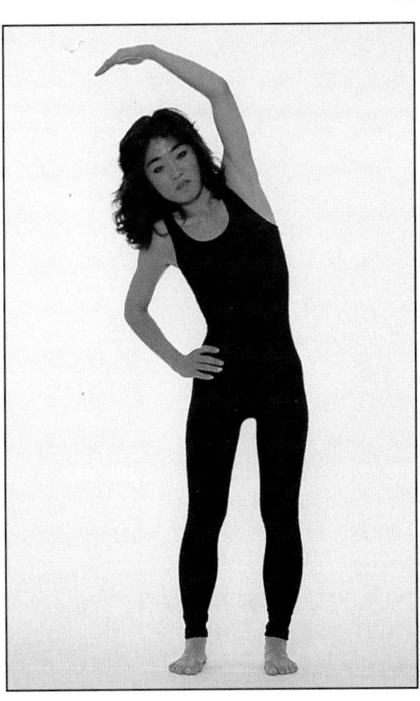

62 Shoulder-and-chest stretch. Stand astride with your arms at shoulder level and elbows bent. Force the elbows backward and return to the starting position. *Repeat 10 times.*

63 Front leg stretch. Stand erect and pull the ankle of one leg to the hip and hold for 20 seconds. Repeat using the other side. *Repeat 10 times.*

64 Side stretch. Bend your trunk to the right with the left arm stretched overhead, then use the same procedure for the other side. *Repeat 10 times.*

B. Weight training

Optimal exercises to increase bone mass and prevent bone loss have not been established. It is clear that the usual aerobic exercises will not accomplish this goal. Strains on the skeleton are best produced by dynamic exercises which may be accomplished using free weights or such machines as Nautilus, Universal, and Omnitron, which are available in most gyms and spas. The majority of gyms retain a professional trainer who is available to devise customized, progressive exercise programmes, and to teach the proper use of equipment. We recommend the programme of weight-lifting such as that demonstrated below. Weight-training exercises use the principles described above of specificity and overload. In addition, progressive resistance must be applied so the work load must be increased from time to time to continue the overload. Exercises are arranged so that progressive exercises do not involve the same muscle groups: thighs and hips, chest and upper arms, back and posterior thighs, legs and arms, back and posterior thighs, legs, and ankles, shoulders and upper arms, abdomen, forearms, wrists. Concepts used in prescribing a dynamic weight-training program include the 'repetition maximum', 'repetitions and set'. The repetition maximum is the greatest weight that can be lifted for a given number of repetitions of an exercise and is a reasonable test of muscle strength. A 'set' consists of the number of consecutive repetitions of the exercise. A typical exercise prescription is three sets done at six repetitions maximum (or 85% per repetition maximum), repeated six times, 6–7 days per week. When ten repetitions can be done the weight is increased. Circuit weight training using low-repetition, high-resistance exercises may prove most beneficial. Such programmes have 6–15 stations. The circuit may be completed many times. There is a 15–20 second rest between stations. Theoretically, it would be preferable for the skeleton to use free weights. A major problem with dynamic weight training is delayed-onset muscle soreness. This may be minimized by using warm-up exercises and progressing gradually.

Exercises for the following regions are shown below: chest and shoulder, **65–70**; upper and lower back, **71–73**; abdomen, **74, 75**; arms, **76, 77**; hips and thighs, **78–83**; and legs, **84**.

65

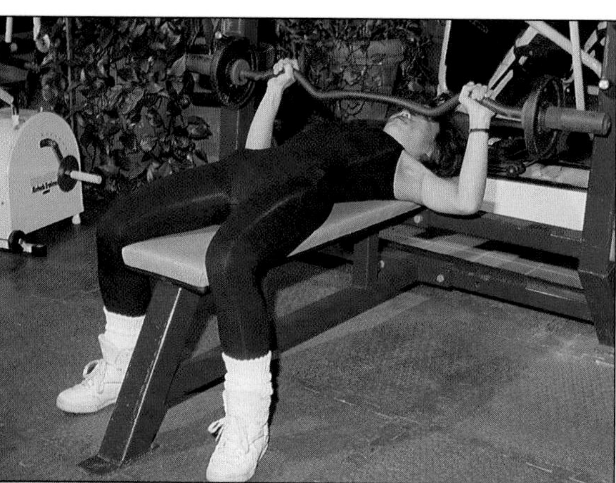

65 Chest and upper arms. *Muscle groups:* shoulder flexors and adductors; elbow extensors. *Equipment:* barbell or bench press station. *Starting position:* (1) pronated (overhand) grip – slightly wider than shoulder-width apart; (2) lying supine on bench, feet on floor astride bench; (3) hold bar at arm's length above chest. *Movement:* (1) lower the bar across chest; (2) vigorously return to starting position.

66

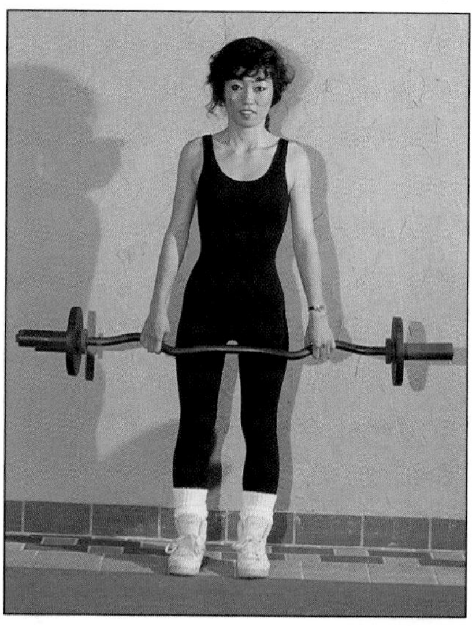

66 Shoulders and upper arms. *Muscle groups:* shoulder girdle elevators. *Equipment:* barbell or bench press station. *Starting position:* (1) pronated grip – slightly wider than shoulder-width apart, forearms extended, legs extended; (2) standing position, bar resting in front of thighs. *Movement:* (1) lift and roll shoulders up and back; (2) return to starting position.

67

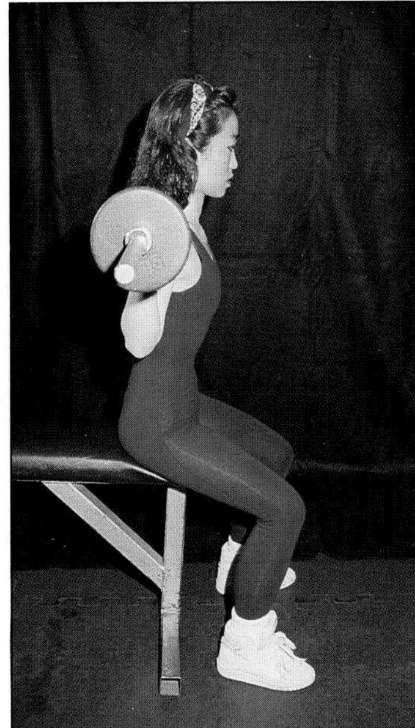

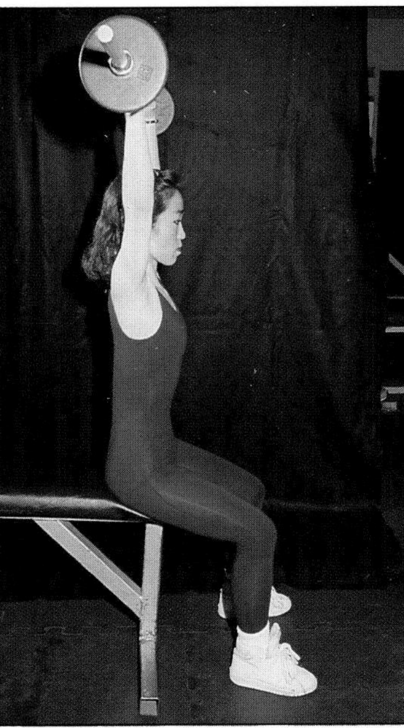

68

67, 68 Chest and upper arms. *Muscle groups:* shoulder flexors and abductors; elbow extensors. *Equipment:* barbell or bench press station. *Starting position:* (1) seated with feet on floor; (2) pronated grip – shoulder-width apart; (3) bar behind head. *Movement:* (1) move the bar to overhead position until elbows are fully extended; (2) return bar to base of neck.

69

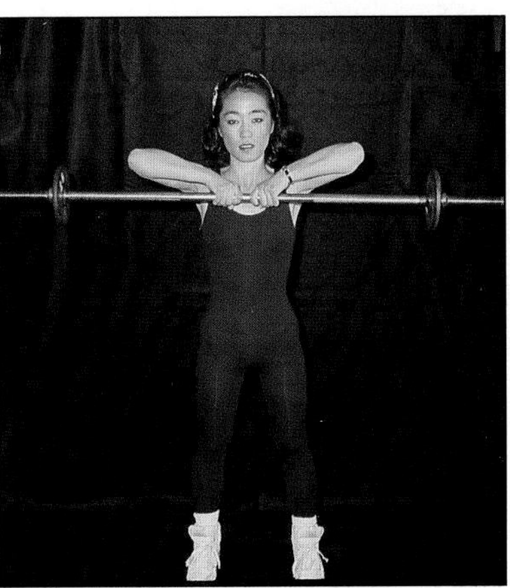

70

69, 70 Shoulders and upper arms. *Muscle groups:* shoulder abductors and elbow flexors. *Equipment:* barbell or curl station. *Starting position:* (1) standing erect, feet apart; (2) overhand grip, hands close together near centre of bar; (3) bar held at waist or hip level. *Movement:* (1) lift bar to chin level; (2) keep elbows high and bar close to body.

71

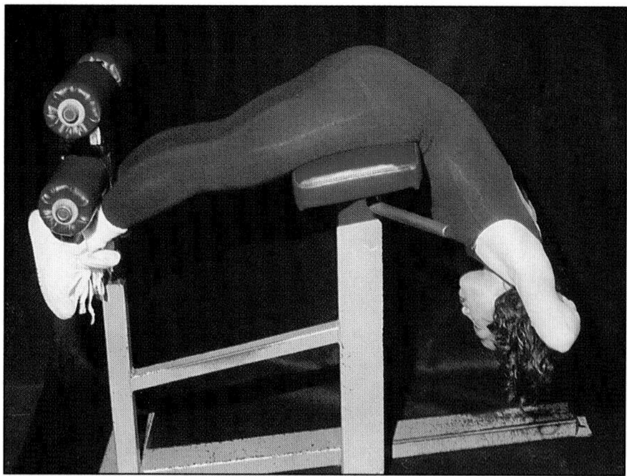

71 Back and posterior thighs. *Muscle groups:* trunk extensors. *Equipment:* trunk lift station. *Starting position:* (1) prone position with trunk unsupported over edge of support and flexed; (2) hands locked behind head. *Movement:* (1) extend trunk so back is parallel to ground; (2) return to starting position.

72

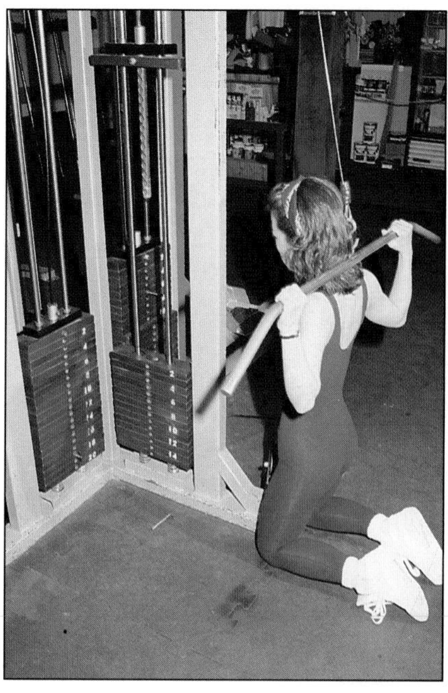

72 Shoulders and upper arms. *Muscle groups:* shoulder extensors and abductors; elbow flexors. *Equipment:* pull-down station. *Starting position:* (1) sitting or kneeling on floor; (2) pronated grip – hands more than shoulder-width apart, elbows extended. *Movement:* (1) pull bar down to base of neck and shoulders; (2) return to starting position.

73

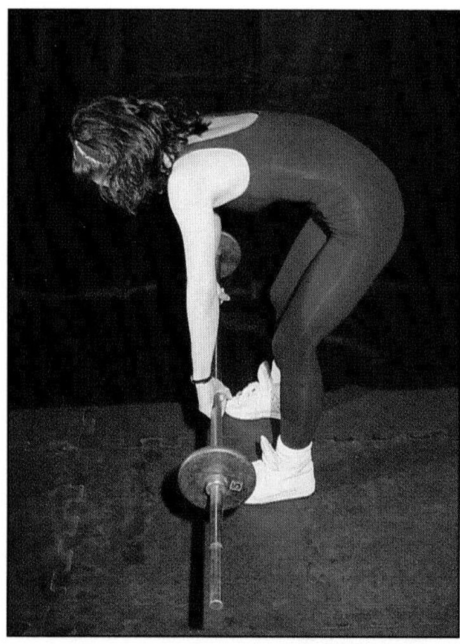

73 Chest and upper arms. *Muscle groups:* shoulder extensors and elbow flexors. *Equipment:* barbell or bench press station. *Starting position:* (1) pronated grip wider than shoulder-width apart; (2) upper trunk parallel to floor, (3) feet spread shoulder-width apart. *Movement:* (1) lift bar up to chest, keeping trunk parallel to floor and knees extended; (2) return to starting position.

74

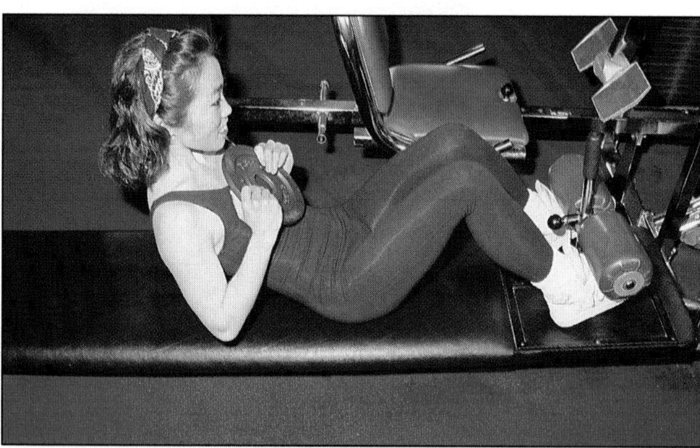

74 Abdomen. *Muscle groups:* trunk flexors and hip flexor. *Equipment:* sit-up station. *Starting position:* (1) supine hook-lying position on incline board; (2) hands and additional weight plates folded across chest. *Movement:* (1) flex trunk to upright sitting position; (2) return to starting position.

75 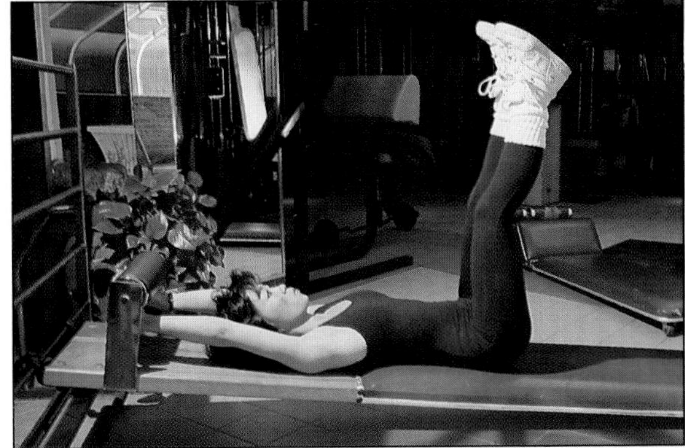

75 Abdomen. *Muscle groups:* hip flexors and lower abdominals. *Equipment:* sit-up station. *Starting position:* (1) lying supine on incline board, knees extended; (2) grasp handle above foot rest. *Movement:* (1) flex hips, keeping legs straight; (2) return to starting position.

76 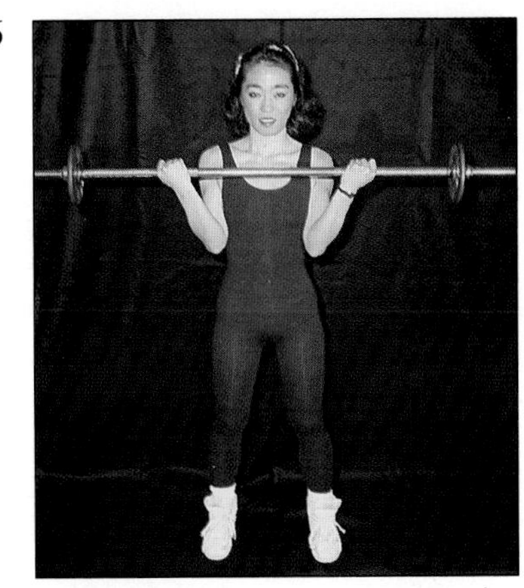

76 Shoulders and upper arms. *Muscle groups*: elbow flexors. *Equipment:* Barbell or curl station. *Starting position*: (1) standing with elbows extended fully and in front of thighs; (2) Supinated grip-shoulder-width apart. *Movement:* (1) flex the elbows, raising bar to chest; do not lean backward; (2) return to starting position.

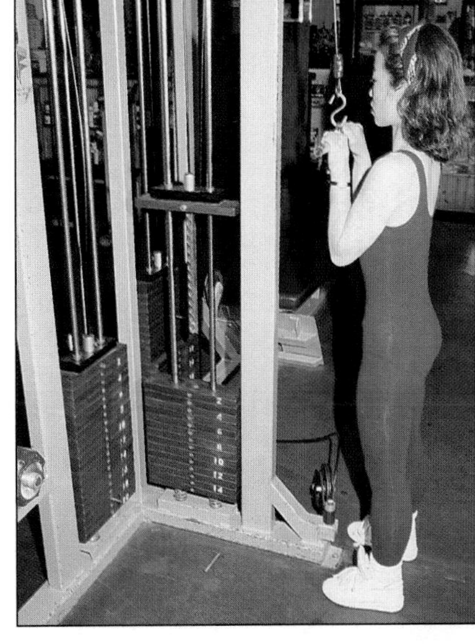 77

77 Shoulders and upper arms. *Muscle groups:* elbow extensors. *Equipment:* pull-down station. *Starting position:* (1) standing with knees extended; (2) pronated grip, hands close together, elbows in close to body, bar about face level. *Movement:* (1) fully extend elbows, pressing bar down; (2) return to starting position.

78 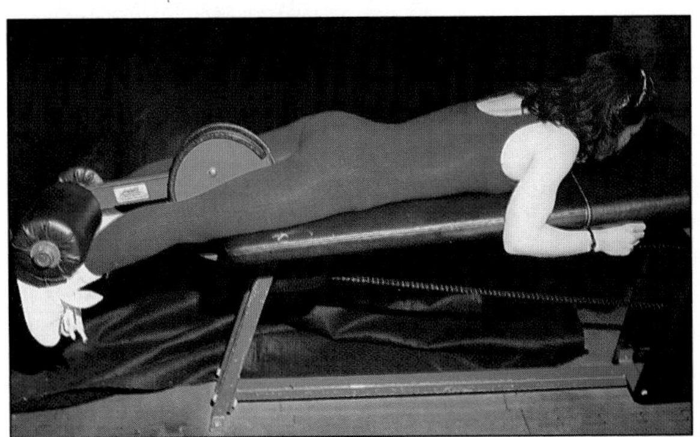

78 Back and posterior thighs. *Muscle groups:* knee flexors. *Equipment:* leg machine. *Starting position:* (1) prone on table, hook heels under support. *Movement:* (1) flex knees, keeping hips flat on table; (2) return to starting position.

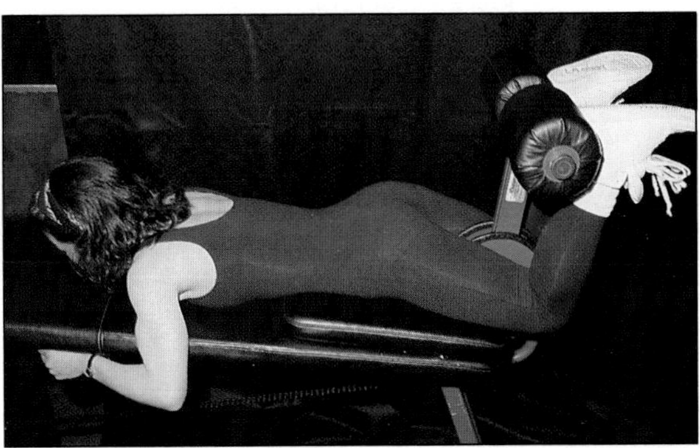 79

79 Legs and ankles. *Muscle groups:* leg extensors. *Equipment:* leg machine. *Starting position:* (1) sitting on end of table with knees flexed at 90°, grasp sides of table; (2) hook ankles under support. *Movement:* (1) fully extend knees, keep trunk erect; (2) return to starting position.

80

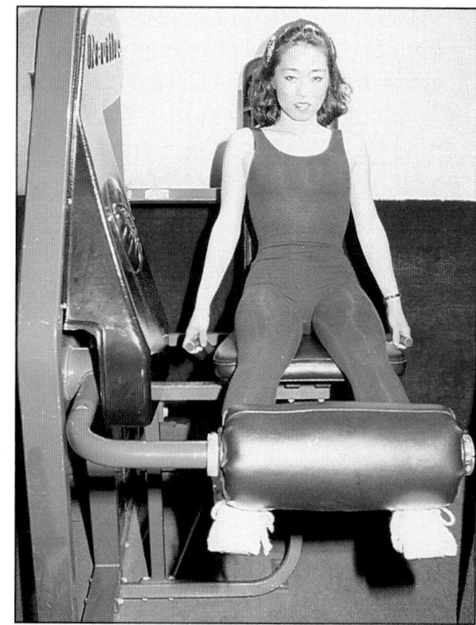

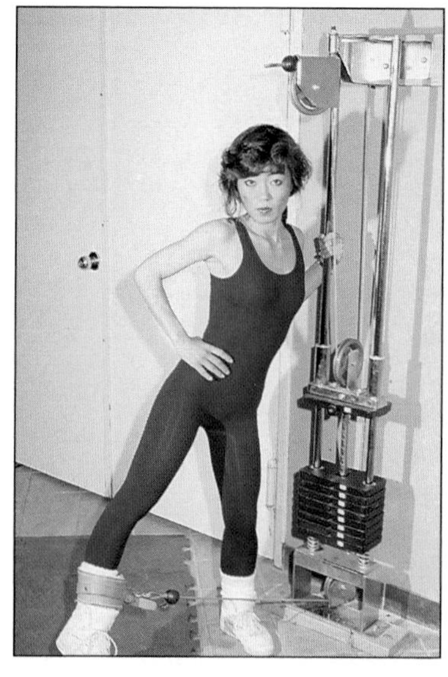

81

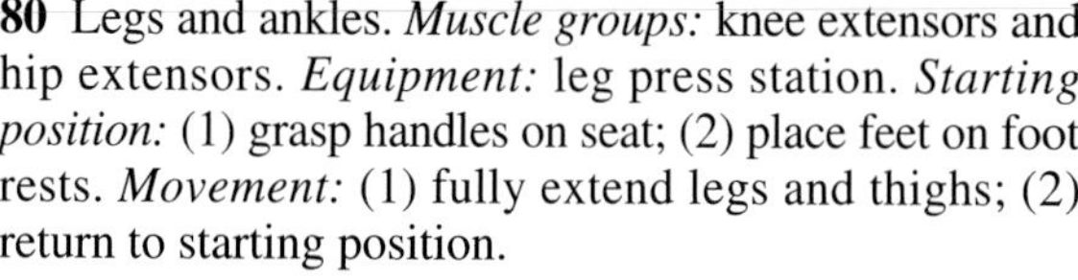

80 Legs and ankles. *Muscle groups:* knee extensors and hip extensors. *Equipment:* leg press station. *Starting position:* (1) grasp handles on seat; (2) place feet on foot rests. *Movement:* (1) fully extend legs and thighs; (2) return to starting position.

81 Thighs and hips. *Muscle groups:* hip abductors or adductors. *Equipment:* pulley station. *Starting position:* (1) standing with side to pulley, hook ankle of either inside leg (for abductors) or outside leg (for adductors) to pulley. *Movement:* (1) fully adduct (abduct) the leg; (2) return to starting position.

82

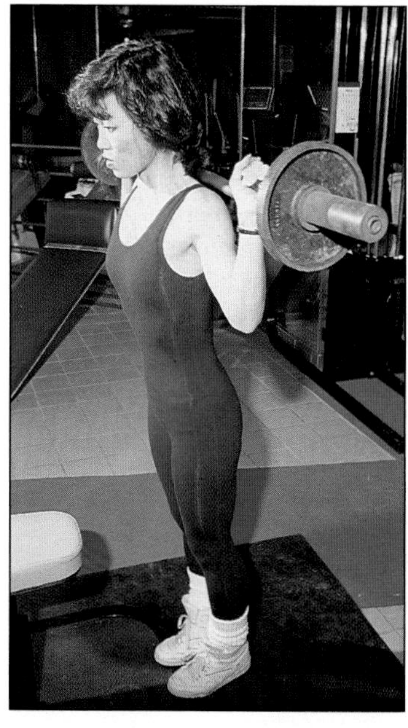

83

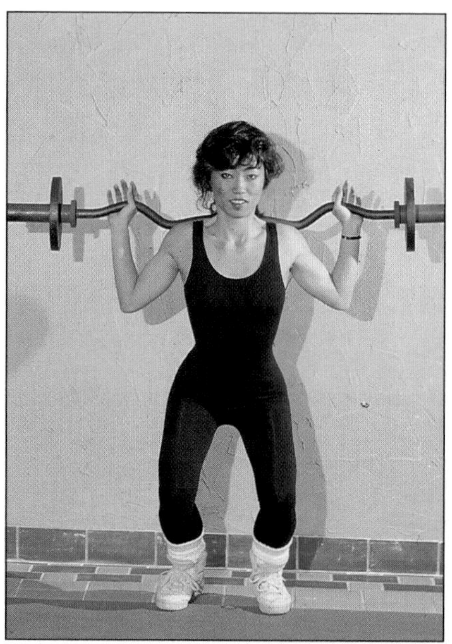

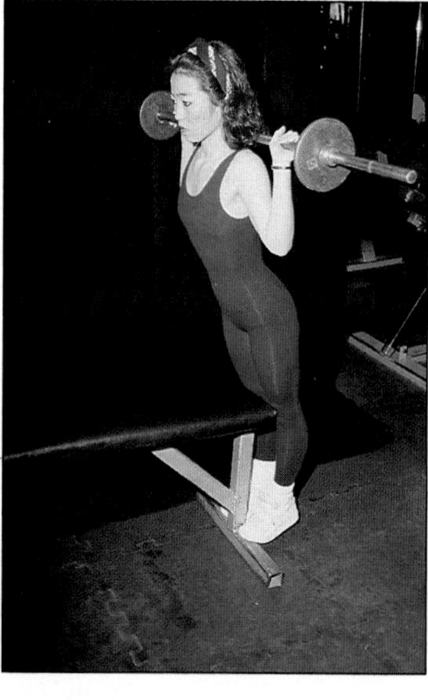

84

82, 83 Thighs and hips. *Muscle groups:* hip, knee, and trunk extensors. *Equipment:* barbell. *Starting position:* (1) standing erect, feet shoulder-width apart, place bar on shoulders behind neck; (2) use pronated grip and spread hands far apart on bar. *Movement:* (1) keeping back straight and head up, lower bar by flexing knees to 90°; (2) return to starting position.

84 Legs and ankles. *Muscle groups:* ankle plantar flexors. *Equipment:* press station or barbell. *Starting position:* (1) standing with balls of feet on board, feet apart, and knees extended; (2) grasp bar shoulder-width apart using pronated grip; rest bar on shoulders. *Movement:* (1) rise up on toes without moving shoulders; (2) return, lowering heels to floor.

C. Aerobic work-out

These exercises should last for 15–20 minutes (**85–88**). They should gradually increase in resistance and duration, with the heart rate being maintained at the target range according to exercise prescriptions.

85

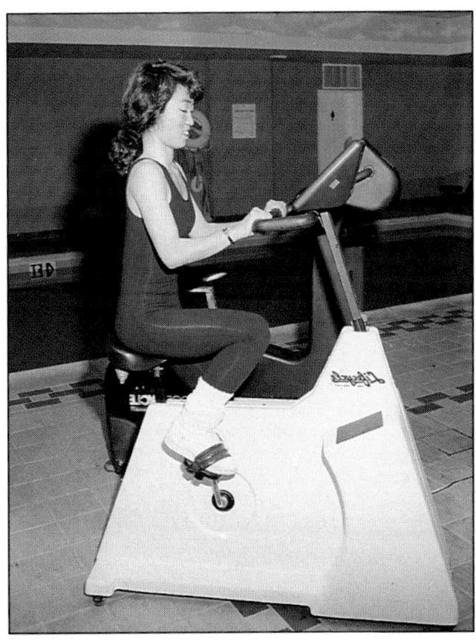

85 Aerobic exercises on a stationary bike.

86

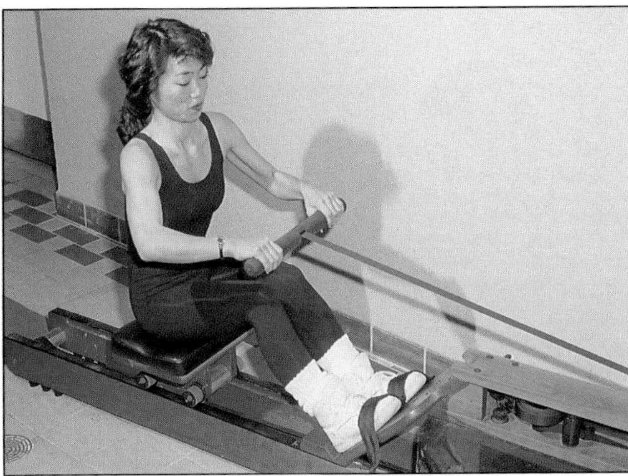

86 Aerobic exercises on a rowing machine.

87

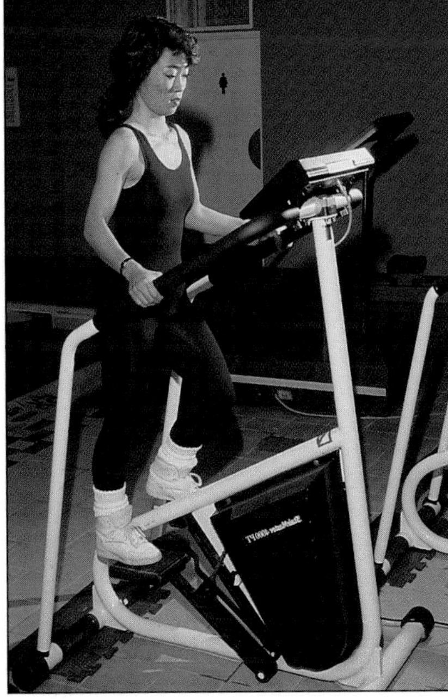

87 Aerobic exercises on a stair-climber.

88

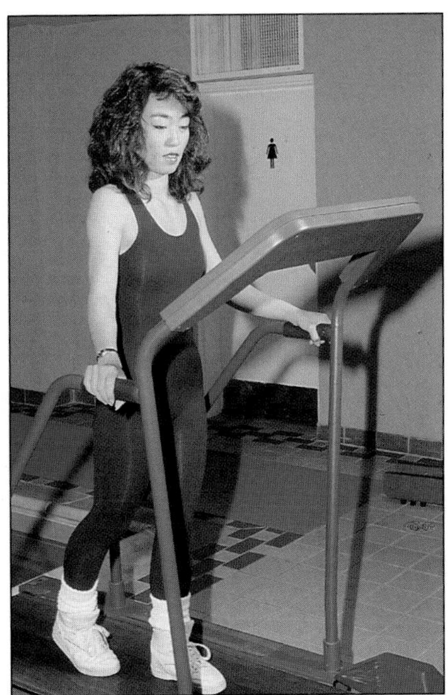

88 Aerobic exercises on a treadmill.

D. Some cool-down exercises

Cool-down with exercises such as those listed previously and sit-ups (**89**), back tighteners (**90, 91**), and back-strengthening exercises (**92**). End up with a T'ai-Chi walk and a practice walk for good posture.

89

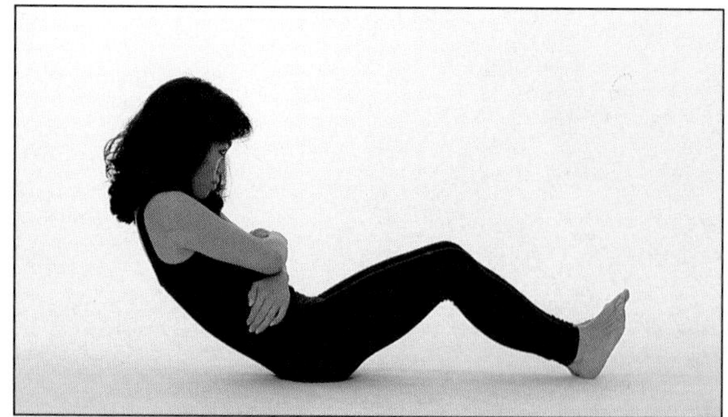

89 Sit-ups as a cool-down exercise.

90

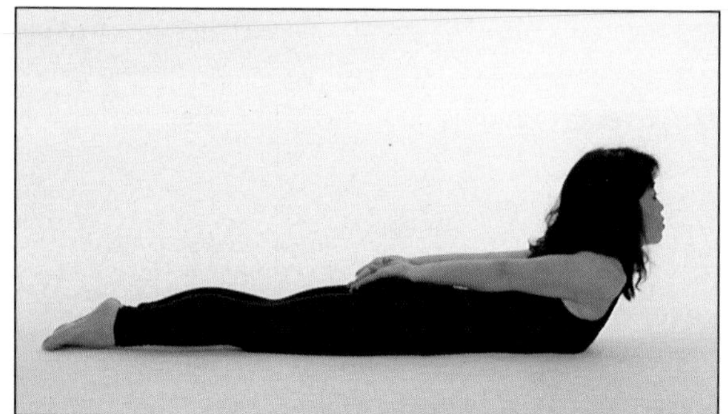

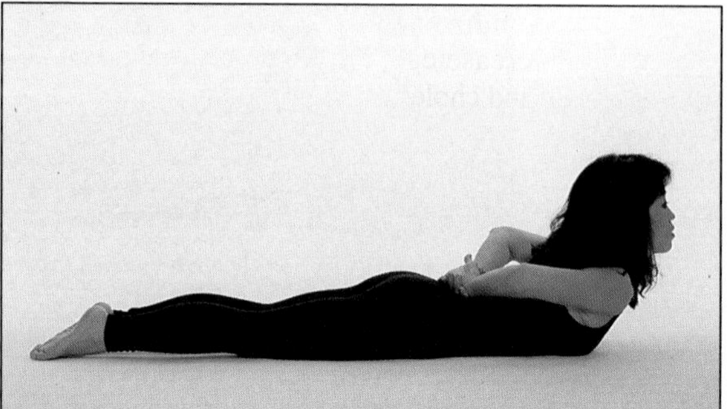

91

90, 91 Back tightners as a cool-down exercise.

92

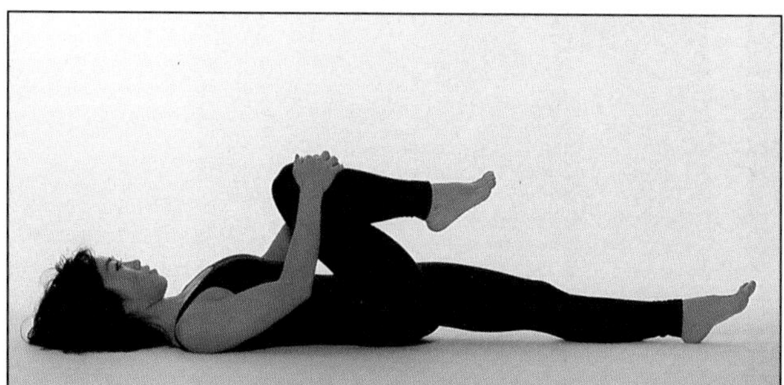

92 Lower back stretch as a cool-down exercise.

4. Prevention through proper nutrition

Introduction

An adequate dietary intake of calcium and vitamin D remains the mainstay of good nutrition in the prevention of osteoporosis. Dairy products are the major source of calcium and vitamin D in western cultures (**93**). Concentration on these products (**94**) will provide adequate intake of calcium. However, optimal nutrition depends on eating a well-balanced diet rather than focusing on one particular nutrient. It would be possible, for instance, to increase calcium intake by adding foods with a high fat and cholesterol content. While the dietary guidelines for Americans may not have applicability in terms of practicality for much of the world they are nonetheless good guidelines for optimal nutrition (**95**). These guidelines will be reviewed here prior to discussion of optimal calcium intake.

93

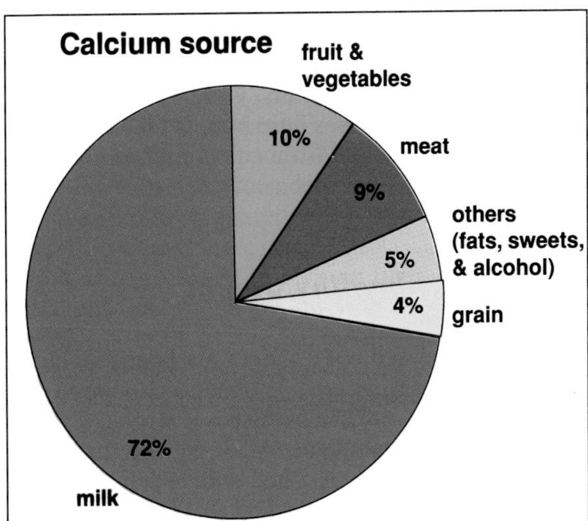

93 The milk group is the primary source of calcium in the American diet.

94

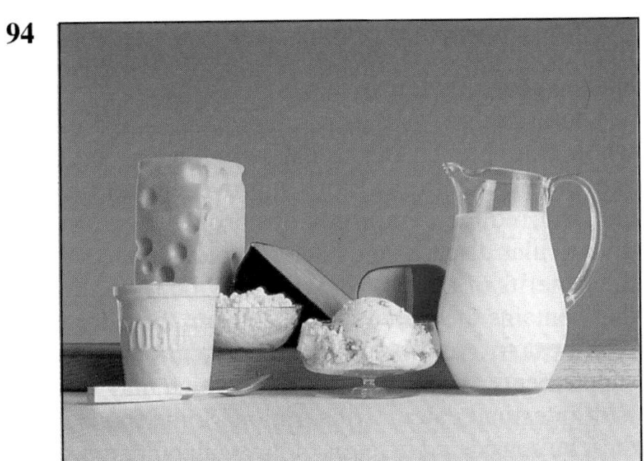

94 Dairy products, a major source of calcium.

95

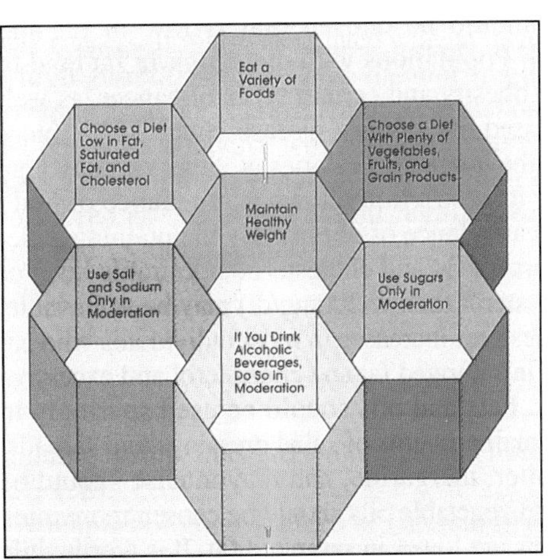

95 Seven dietary guidelines for Americans.

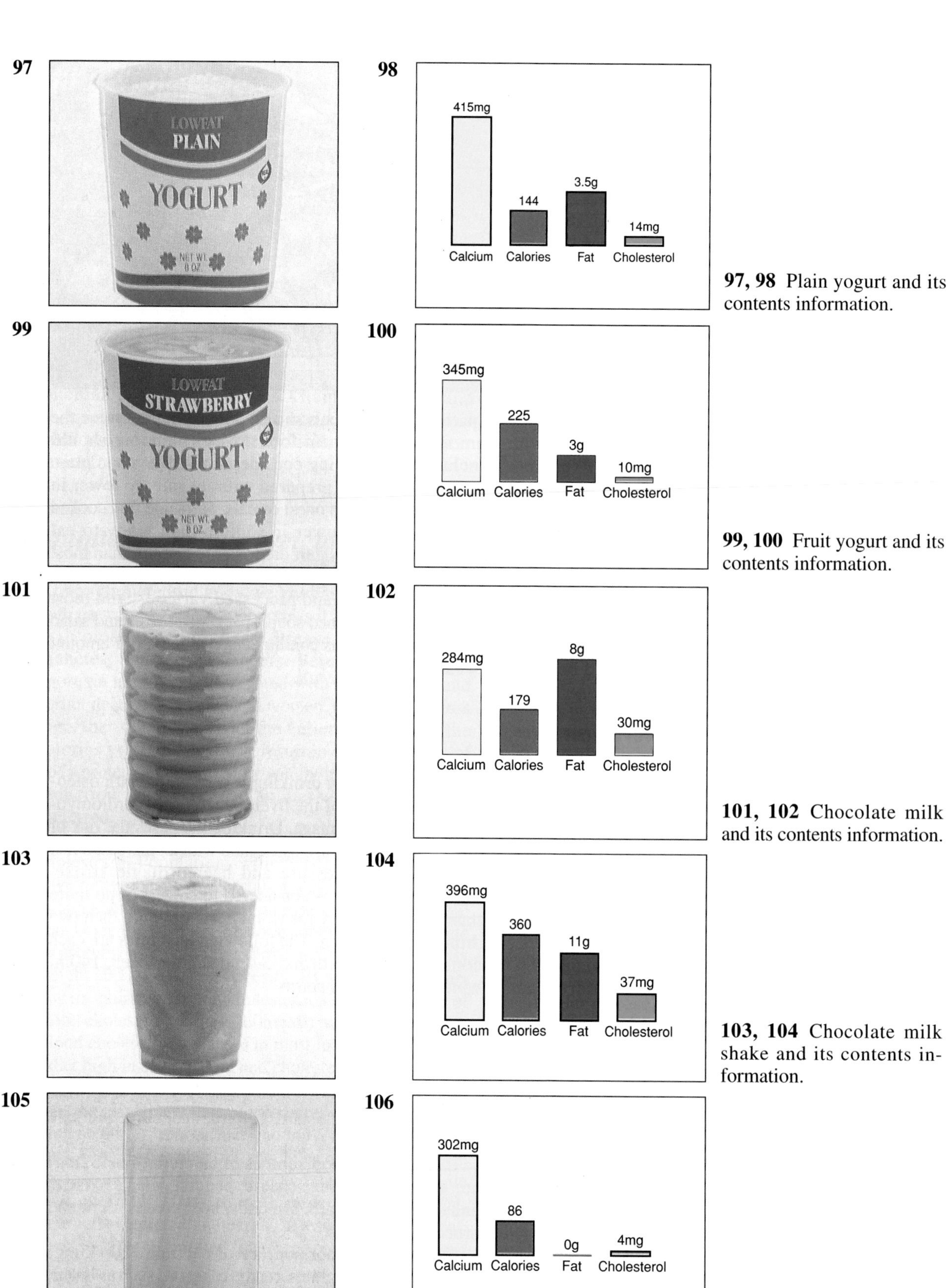

97, 98 Plain yogurt and its contents information.

99, 100 Fruit yogurt and its contents information.

101, 102 Chocolate milk and its contents information.

103, 104 Chocolate milk shake and its contents information.

105, 106 Skimmed milk and its contents information.

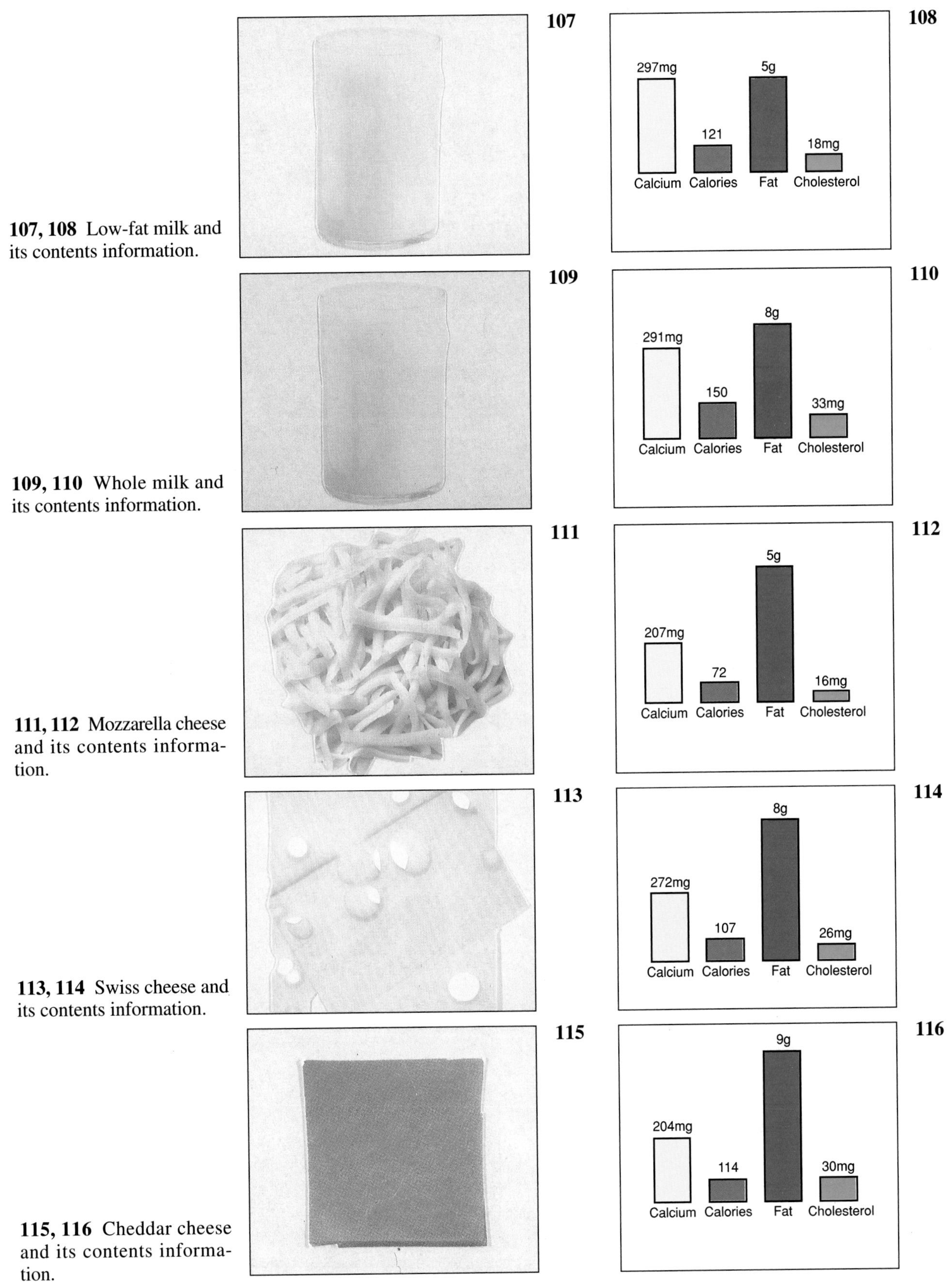

107, 108 Low-fat milk and its contents information.

109, 110 Whole milk and its contents information.

111, 112 Mozzarella cheese and its contents information.

113, 114 Swiss cheese and its contents information.

115, 116 Cheddar cheese and its contents information.

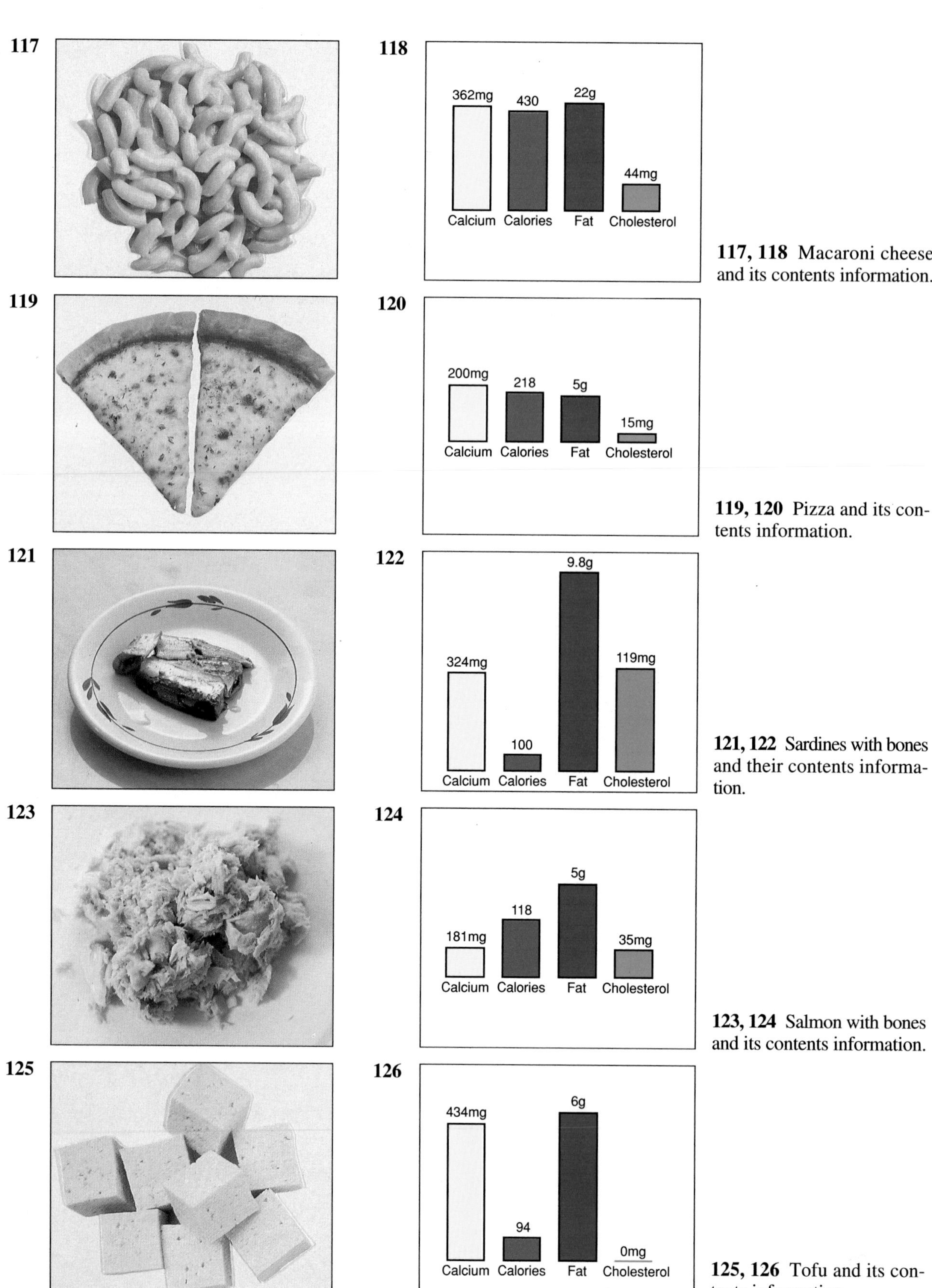

117, 118 Macaroni cheese and its contents information.

119, 120 Pizza and its contents information.

121, 122 Sardines with bones and their contents information.

123, 124 Salmon with bones and its contents information.

125, 126 Tofu and its contents information.

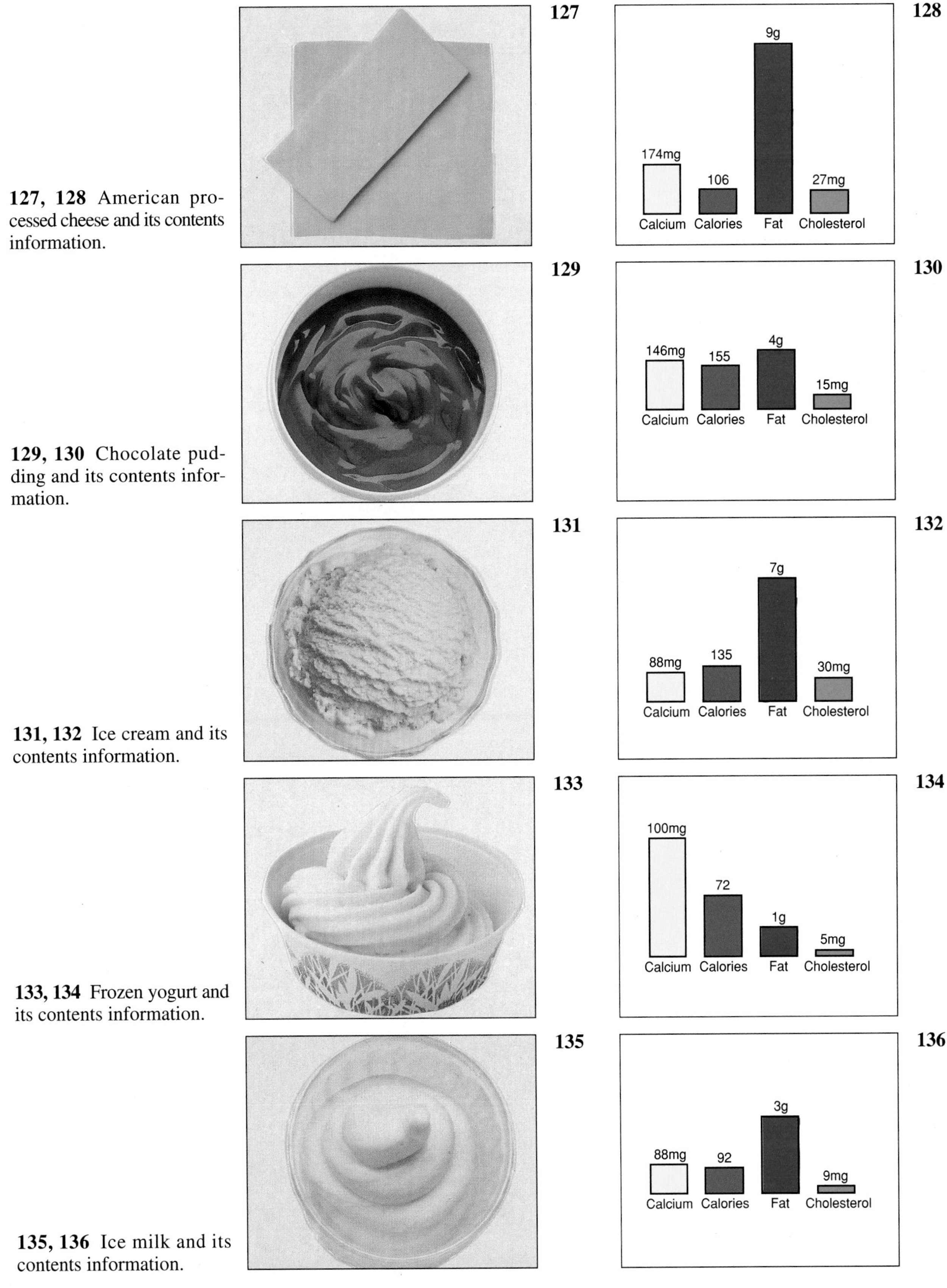

127, 128 American processed cheese and its contents information.

129, 130 Chocolate pudding and its contents information.

131, 132 Ice cream and its contents information.

133, 134 Frozen yogurt and its contents information.

135, 136 Ice milk and its contents information.

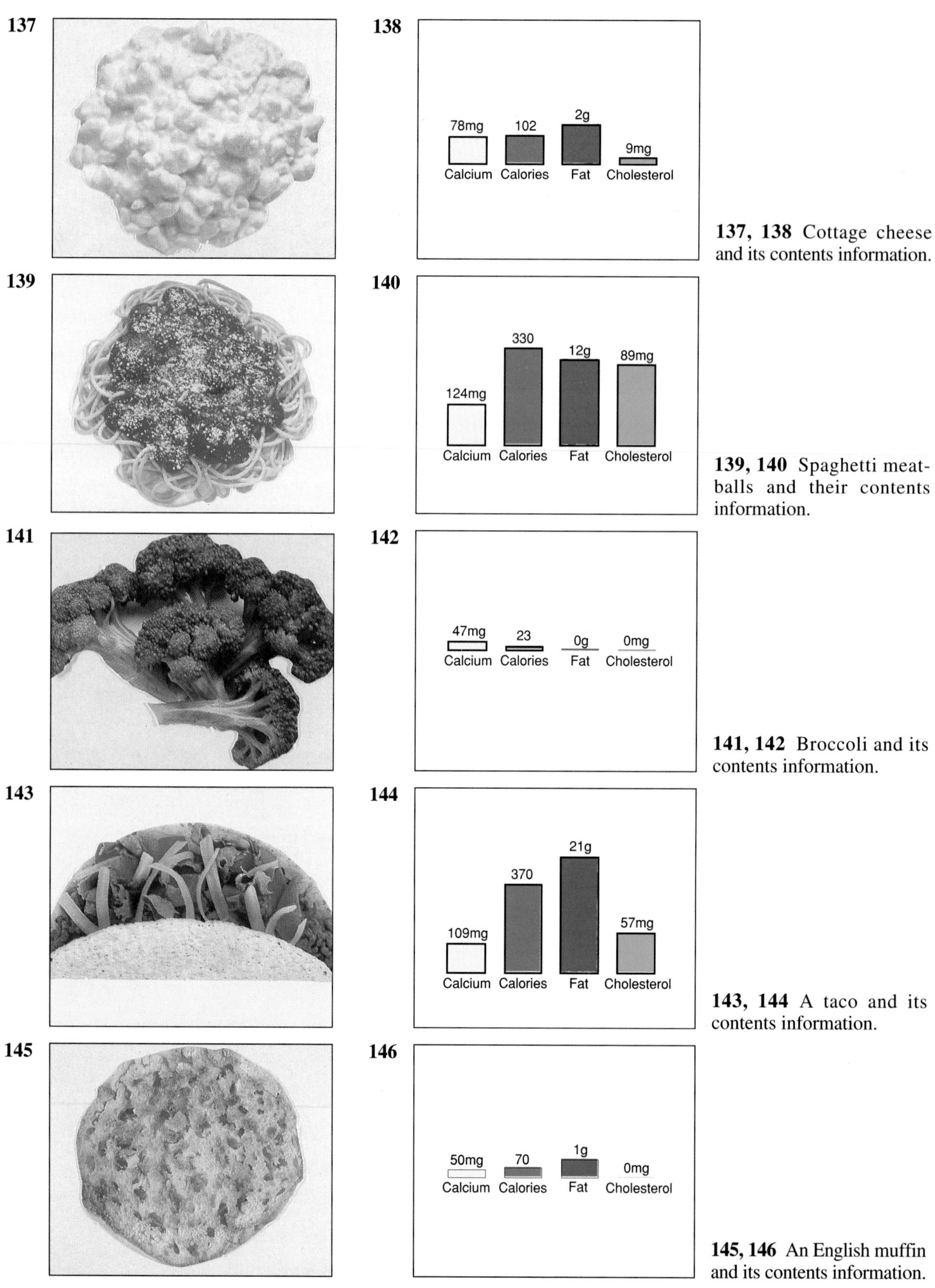

137, 138 Cottage cheese and its contents information.

139, 140 Spaghetti meatballs and their contents information.

141, 142 Broccoli and its contents information.

143, 144 A taco and its contents information.

145, 146 An English muffin and its contents information.

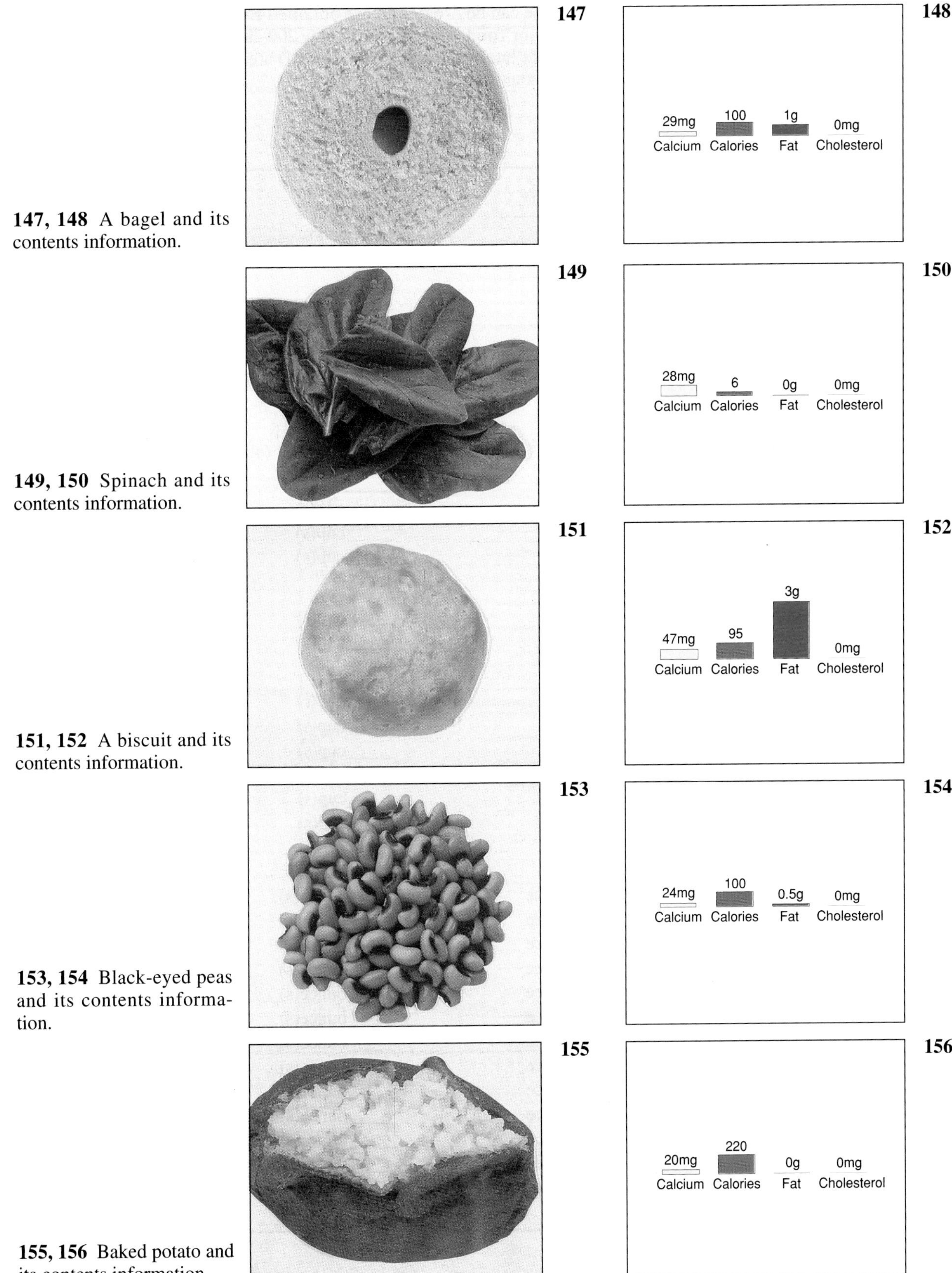

147, 148 A bagel and its contents information.

149, 150 Spinach and its contents information.

151, 152 A biscuit and its contents information.

153, 154 Black-eyed peas and its contents information.

155, 156 Baked potato and its contents information.

Table 16. Food sources of vitamin D.

Food	*Amount*	*Vitamin D (μg)*
Dairy Products		
Milk, whole, low-fat, or skimmed fortified with vitamin D	8 ounces	100
Cheese, Swiss (Emmentaler)	3½ ounces	100
Egg, yolk	1	60
Butter	1 tablespoon	6
Cream, heavy	1 tablespoon	6
Fish		
Eel, smoked	3½ ounces	6,400
Eel, unsmoked	3½ ounces	5,000
Herring	3½ ounces	900
Salmon, Atlantic	3½ ounces	650
Salmon, Atlantic, canned with solids and liquids	3½ ounces	500
Sardines, canned in oil, drained solids	3½ ounces	250
Shrimp, canned, drained solids	3½ ounces	105
Mackerel	3½ ounces	50
Oysters	3½ ounces	5
Liver		
Liver, calf or chicken	3½ ounces	50
Oils		
Cod liver oil	1 tablespoon	1,215
Other		
Mushrooms	3½ ounces	150

Since many women still have less than 400mg/day of calcium in their diet, it is necessary to make significant changes in dietary habits to achieve a daily intake of 1,000 or 1,500mg . Seventy-two percent of the available calcium in the American diet comes from dairy products. Tofu, one of the non-dairy products high in calcium, is also high in protein but relatively low in fat: its saturated fat content is lower than that of chicken and its cholesterol content is zero. As discussed previously, green leafy vegetables may have a high calcium content, but they may also have low bio-availability and should not be used as calcium sources. Meat and poultry products are poor sources of calcium – with the exception of alligator meat. Cereals (unless enriched) and most fruits and juices are low in calcium. A variety of food choices may be chosen to increase the calcium content of the diet. There are dozens of calcium-fortified foods available; for example, low-fat milk with added calcium, breads with natural calcium enrichment, calcium-fortified flour, and orange juice fortified with 300mg of calcium citrate malate per cup.

There are many recommended ways of increasing dietary calcium intake. They include: eating more tofu, dairy products and fortified foods; preparing soup stock with the bones of meat with added vinegar to draw the calcium out of the bones; adding milk or non-fat dry milk to soups; adding powdered non-fat dry milk to hot beverages and soups as well as to cake, bread and cookie recipes; using non-fat milk in cooking wherever possible; and adding cheese chunks or shredded cheese to salads, vegetables, soups, sandwiches, and meat. Ideally, each meal should contain a high calcium food, and snacks throughout the day should consist of dairy products such as skimmed milk or yogurt. Attention must be paid to the fat and cholesterol content of calcium-rich foods. Compare and contrast the fat, calorie and cholesterol levels of the various calcium rich foods. Note, for example, the difference between skimmed and whole milk (**106** and **110**).

Sample menus

It requires some thought to increase calcium intake without also increasing caloric intake. **157–168** show menus with different total calorie intake and calcium content. Because men have a higher caloric intake than women they may find it easier to increase their calcium intake without weight gain.

157

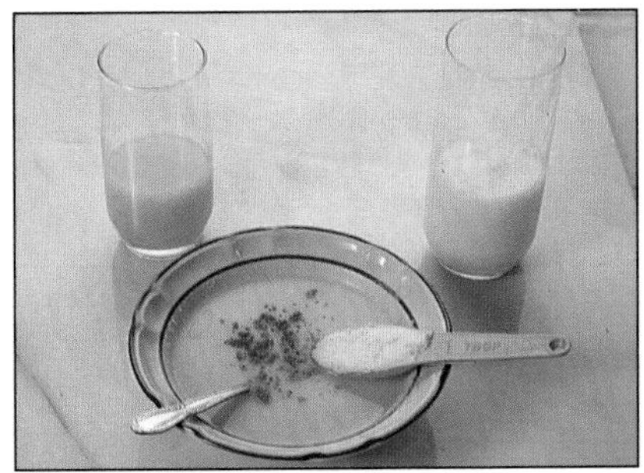

158

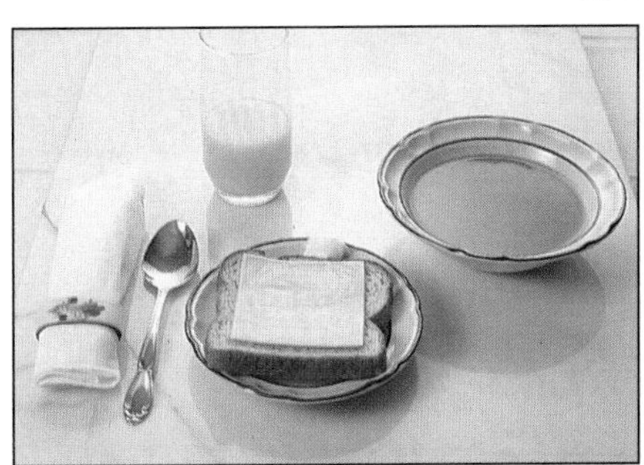

157–160 A suggested day's menu containing 1,200mg of calcium and having a total of 1,200 calories: **157**, breakfast (porridge and milk); **158**, lunch (bread, cheese and tomato soup); **159**, dinner (baked potato, carrots, grilled meat, fruit and milk); and **160**, a snack (yogurt).

159

160

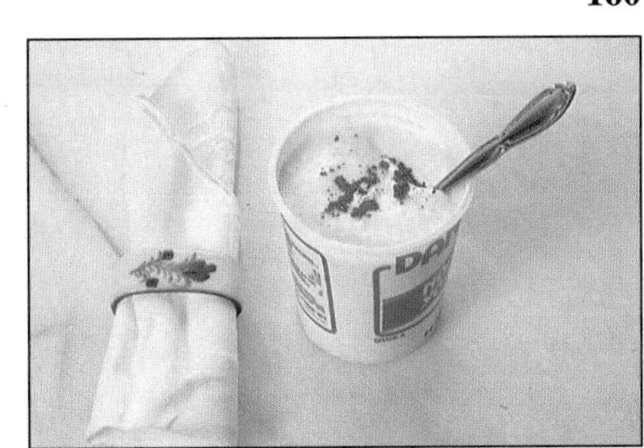

161

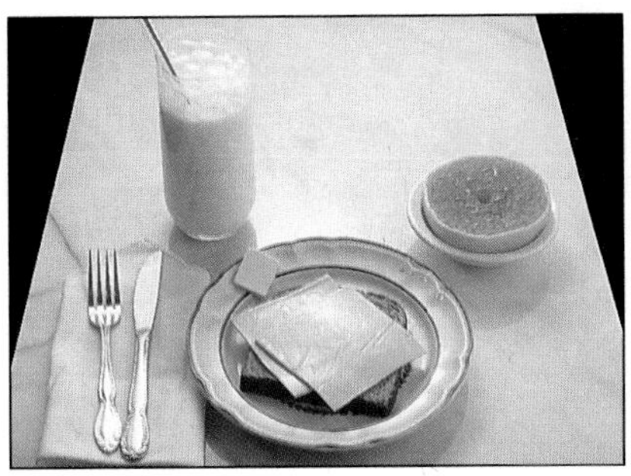

162

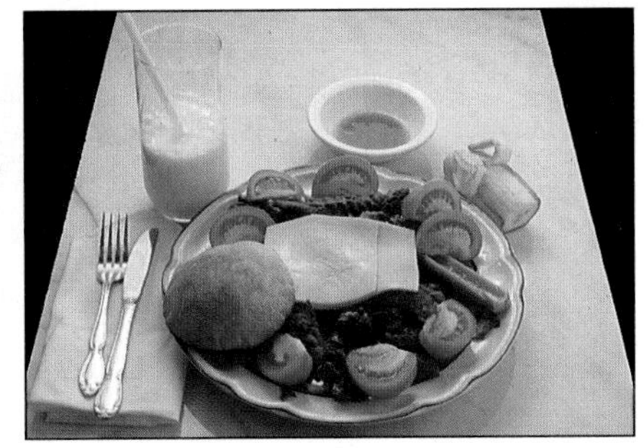

161–164 A suggested day's menu containing 1,500mg of calcium and having a total of 1,200 calories: **161**, breakfast (bread, butter, cheese, milk and grapefruit); **162**, lunch (wholewheat pita bread, cheese, celery, tomatoes,oil and vinegar, banana, and milk); **163**, dinner (pork, green beans, butter, cabbage, mashed potato, an apple and milk); and **164**, a snack (chocolate pudding).

163

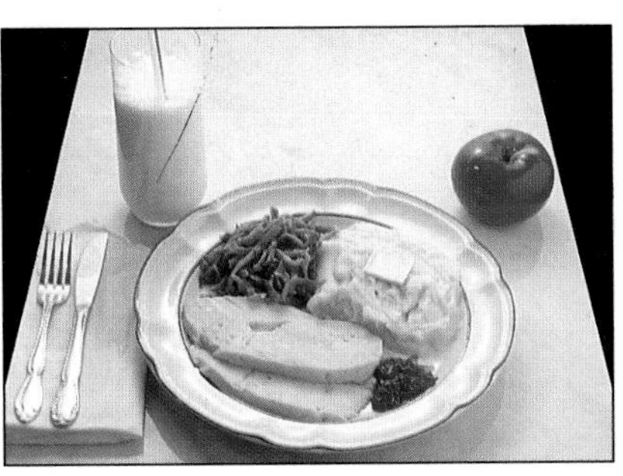

164

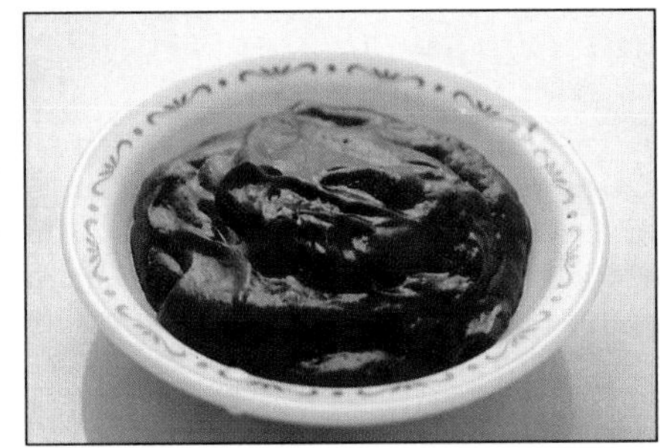

165

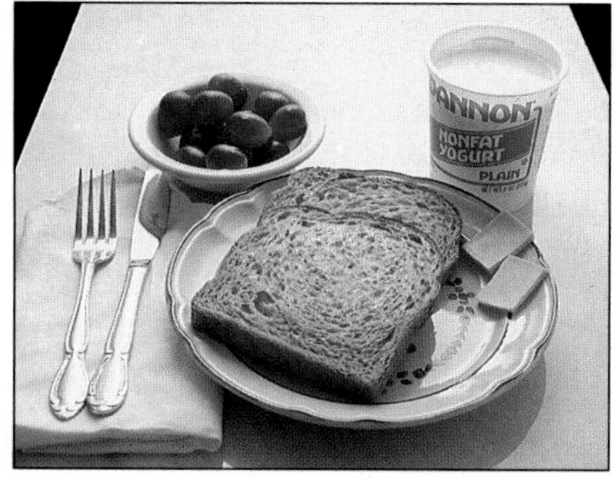

166

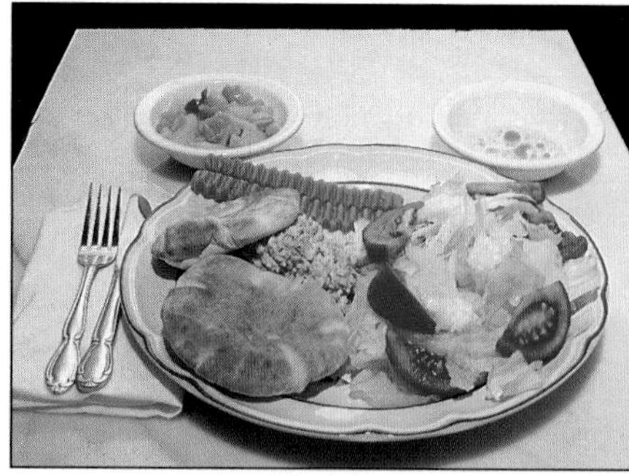

167

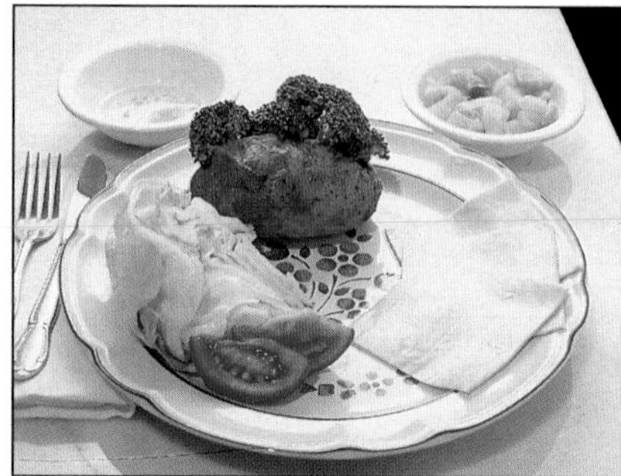

168

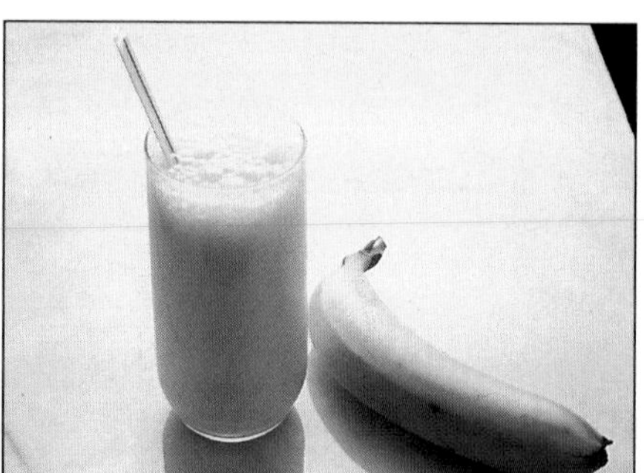

165–168 A suggested day's menu containing 1,500mg of calcium and having a total of 1,800 calories: **165**, breakfast (wholewheat bread, butter, yogurt and grapes); **166**, lunch (pitta bread, salad, carrot, salmon and fruit); **167**, dinner (baked potato, salad, oil and vinegar, cheese and fruit); and **168**, a snack (milk shake and a banana).

The Recommended Daily Allowance

169

Percentage of U.S.
Recommended Daily Allowances (U.S. RDA)

PROTEIN	20	VITAMIN D	25
VITAMIN A	10	VITAMIN B6	4
VITAMIN C	4	VITAMIN B12	15
THIAMINE	6	PHOSPHORUS	20
RIBOFLAVIN	25	MAGNESIUM	8
NIACIN	*	ZINC	4
CALCIUM	30	PANTOTHENIC ACID	6
IRON	*		

*Contains less than 2% of the U.S. RDA of these nutrients.
INGREDIENTS: LOWFAT MILK (2% MILKFAT) WITH VITAMIN A PALMITATE AND 400 I.U. VITAMIN D2 ADDED PER QUART.

The Recommended Daily Allowance is a set of standards developed in the United States by the Food and Drug Administration for the purpose of regulating the nutritional labelling of food (**169**). This is useful in shopping. The RDA (Recommended Dietary Allowance) may have different values.

169 A food label from a carton of low-fat milk.

Calcium supplements

Despite the media blitz that resulted in the 'calcium craze' where many women believed that increasing calcium intake alone could prevent osteoporosis, the average intake of menopausal women in the United States remains in the range of about 500mg per day.

Sales of calcium supplements in the United States exceeded $200,000,000 in 1987, with a confusing array of supplements available to the consumer. In addition to being a factor in the reduction of bone loss, a high calcium intake has been thought to be protective against cancer of the colon, hypertension, and periodontal disease. While it is clear that the pathogenesis of osteoporosis is multi-factorial, an adequate dietary calcium intake should be provided. However, many women will not adequately increase their food intake to accomplish this goal. Calcium supplementations have varied bioavailability. Some of them are not readily dissolved. Of course, calcium is not present in the free form but is combined with other substances. Calcium carbonate is obtained from oyster shell or egg shell. Bone meal and dolomite are not recommended as calcium sources because they contain other substances that may be harmful. Calcium gluconate has few undesirable side effects. Calcium glubionate is available (in liquid form for those who do not want to swallow or chew tablets). Calcium citrate has the advantage of being absorbed when gastric acid secretion is a problem. In addition, the citrate form is protective against the formation of calcium-rich kidney stones.

Of course, anyone with any form of kidney disease should be evaluated prior to increasing their calcium intake. Calcium citrate malate has been suggested in one study to be most effective in preventing bone loss, but is currently only available as a food supplement. To increase patient compliance it is generally desirable to use calcium compounds with a high percentage of their weight being comprised of calcium *(Table 17)*. If calcium carbonate is prescribed for the elderly or anyone who may have decreased gastric acid secretion it should be given with meals.

A simplified approach to calcium intake is preferable. Individuals should include 300mg or 500mg of calcium-supplying foods (see *Tables 18* and *19*) in each meal and as a bedtime snack, depending on the dietary goal. If this is not possible at any meal, a calcium supplement should be substituted. There is insufficient information to apply to any individual to warrant obsessive concern over 100mg differences in daily calcium intake

Table 17. Elemental calcium content of various sources.

Calcium source	*Percentage of elemental calcium*
Calcium carbonate	40
Calcium sulphate	36
Tribasic calcium phosphate	39
Bone meal	32
Dibasic calcium phosphate	29
Dolomite	22
Calcium lactate	13
Calcium ascorbate	10
Calcium gluconate	9
Calcium glubionate	6.5
Calcium citrate	24
Calcium citrate malate	24

Table 18. Quantities of foods containing approximately 300mg calcium.

Milk—8 ounces
Swiss cheese—1 1/4 ounces
Cottage cheese—2 cups
Cheddar cheese—1 1/2 ounces
Yogurt, fruited—1 cup
Ice cream—1 1/2 cups
Custard—1 cup
Alba Hi-Calcium beverage—8 ounces
Home-made macaroni and cheese—3/4 cup
Tofu—1 cup
Almonds—3/4 cup
Cheese pizza—2 slices
Sardines—6–7 medium
Salmon (canned, with bones)—5 ounces
Calcium carbonate—750mg

Table 19. Quantities of food containing approximately 500mg of calcium.

Milk—14 ounces	Custard—1 2/3 cups
Calcimilk (fortified milk)—8 ounces	Home-made macaroni and cheese—1 1/4 cups
Vanilla milkshake—12 ounces	Tofu—1 3/4 cups
Swiss cheese—2 1/4 ounces	Cheese pizza—3 slices
Cottage cheese—3 1/3 cups	Sardines—11 medium
Cheddar cheese—2 1/2 ounces	Salmon (canned, with bones)—9 ounces
Yogurt, plain, low-fat—10 ounces	Calcium carbonate—1250mg
Ice cream—2 3/4 cups	

5. Secondary osteoporoses

Introduction

Osteoporosis may be considered to be primary or secondary to a diagnosable underlying illness. Indeed, primary osteoporosis is diagnosed by exclusion of any of the secondary disorders. A classification of osteoporosis is given in *Tables 20* and *21*. Although we have concentrated on osteoporosis in women one-seventh of all vertebral compression fractures and a quarter of all hip fractures occur in men. Osteoporosis is less common in men because of their higher peak bone mass, their shorter life expectancy, and the lack of menopausal bone loss. When osteoporosis in men occurs in their fifties or sixties, there is more likely to be an identifiable underlying cause than in women. Thus, for men, it is especially important to exclude the secondary causes of osteoporosis described below. A male with idiopathic osteoporosis is shown in **170**. Risk factors for osteoporosis in men are thought to include Caucasian ancestry, immobilization, inactivity, delayed puberty, hypogonadism, alcoholism, glucocorticoid use, dietary calcium deficiency, cigarette smoking, and gastric or intestinal surgery. In younger males with idiopathic osteoporosis, i.e, when a secondary cause is not known, it is common for bone remodelling to be evaluated. Juvenile osteoporosis is osteoporosis developing in prepubertal boys and girls (**171**). The osteoporosis is accompanied by fractures and disability for 2–4 years.

Table 20. Classification of primary osteoporosis.

Juvenile
Idiopathic
Postmenopausal
Involutional

170

171

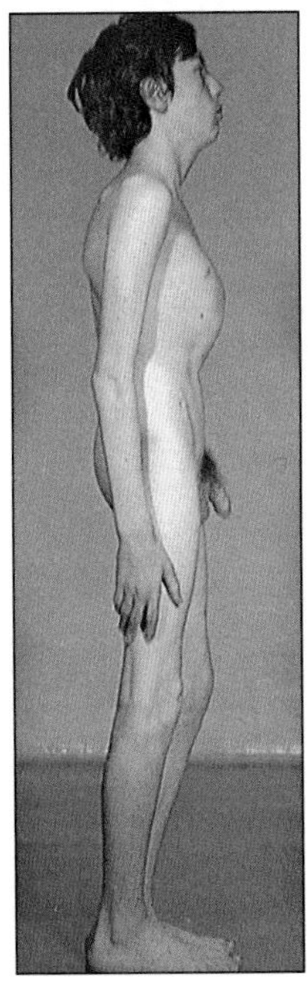

170 A male with idiopathic osteoporosis.

171 Juvenile osteoporosis.

Table 21. Possible causes of secondary osteopoenia.

Congenital	
Osteogenesis imperfecta	Hypophosphatasia
Homocystinuria	Haemolytic anaemia
Endocrine	
Prolactinaemia	Hypogonadism
Cushing's syndrome	Hyperparathyroidism
Growth hormone deficiency	Type I diabetes mellitus
Hyperthyroidism	
Drugs	
Glucocorticoids	Alcohol
Anticonvulsants	GnRH antagonists or agonists
Methotrexate	Thyrotoxicosis factitia
Loop diuretics	
Heparin	
Diet	
Calcium deficiency	Starvation (anorexia)
Scurvy	
Miscellaneous	
Renal tubular acidosis	Rheumatoid arthritis
Immobilization	Mastocytosis
Liver disease	Multiple myeloma
Lymphoma	Leukaemia
Haemolytic anaemia	Alcoholism
Malabsorption	GI surgery

Following this, a spontaneous remission usually occurs followed by resumption of bone growth. Idiopathic osteoporosis occurs in postpubertal adults, and is characterized by vertebral fractures, although fractures of the ribs and long bones may also occur. The clinical course of this disorder may be mild but it is more often very severe and rapidly progressive.

Involutional osteoporosis has been sub-categorized into Type I (postmenopausal) and Type II (senescent) osteoporosis. The characteristics of these two types of osteoporosis are given in *Table 22*. Type I, or postmenopausal osteoporosis, affects women up to 15–20 years after menopause. This disorder was originally described in 1941 by Fuller Albright and his associates. Vertebral compression fractures and Colles' fracture are mainly observed. The vertebral fractures are mostly associated with extreme deformation and pain. It is believed that women with Type I osteoporosis have lost an excessive amount of trabecular bone (**172**). The mechanisms proposed for the pathogenesis of Type I osteoporosis are linked to menopause which results in accelerated bone loss, transient hypercalcaemia, decreased secretion of parathyroid hormone, decreased formation of calcitriol, and subsequent decreased calcium absorption. The decrease in parathyroid hormone levels is thought to be due to the increased bone resorption which results from oestrogen withdrawal. Other investigators believe that oestrogen withdrawal produces hypercalciuria which results in secondary hyperparathyroidism. The inability of the postmenopausal woman to augment intestinal calcium absorption then leads to bone loss (**173**). In Type II osteoporosis (called senile osteoporosis by Albright) the age group is over 70 years; this type occurs in both men and women (**174**). It is manifested mainly by hip and vertebral fractures, although fractures of the foot, humerus, rib, toe, leg, pelvis, hand, and clavicle are related to reduced bone mass. (Fractures of the ankle, elbow, finger, and face are not associated with low bone mass.) The vertebral fractures are often of the multiple wedge type leading to dorsal kyphosis. The vertebral deformation may be painless. One factor in the development of involutional osteoporosis in addition to aging is the reduced renal production of calcitriol which

Table 22. Postmenopausal (Type I) and involutional (Type II) osteoporosis.

Factors	*Type I*	*Type II*
Age	55–75	>70
Sex (F:M)	6:1	2:1
Fracture types	Wrist/vertebrae	Hip/vertebrae, long bones
Hormonal cause	Oestrogen deficiency	Calcitriol deficiency
Calcium absorption	Decreased	Decreased
Increased parathyroid hormone	No	Yes
Importance of dietary calcium	Moderate	High

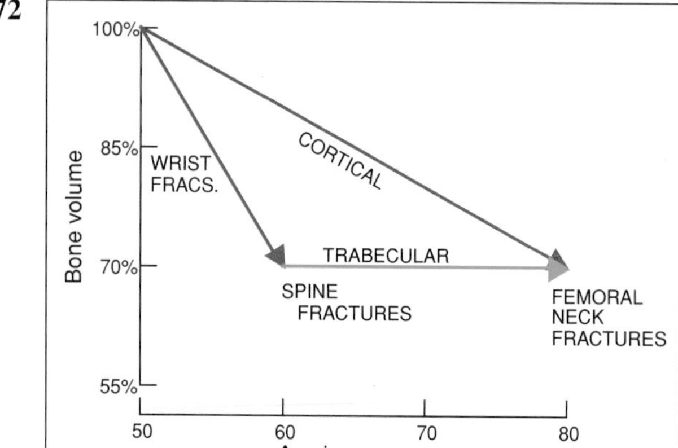

172 Graph showing different bone volume losses with age.

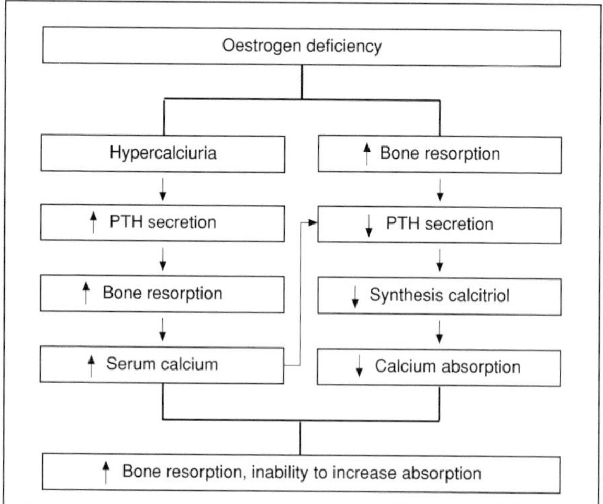

173 A diagram showing two postulates of pathogenesis of Type I osteoporosis, both involving parathyroid hormone (PTH).

174

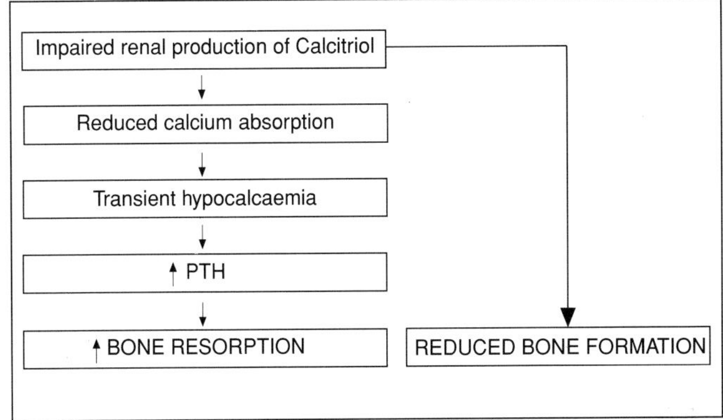

174 A diagram showing the proposed pathogensis of Type II osteoporosis.

175

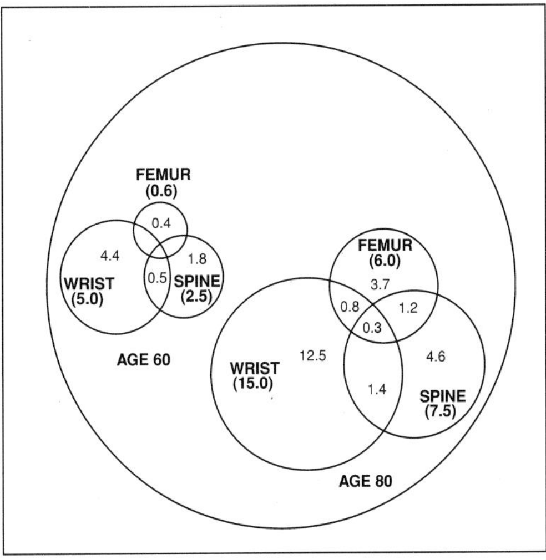

175 Types of fractures in the female population as a percentage.

results in decreased calcium absorption and secondary hyperparathyroidism. The types of fractures in Type I and Type II osteoporosis are shown in **175**.

While this classification may have some clinical utility, it is important to realize that osteoporosis is multifactorial in aetiology. Moreover, rather than two distinct clinical syndromes, there appears to be a significant overlap between Types I and II osteoporosis, suggesting a continuum. Histomorphometric analysis of bone biopsies in osteoporotic women with spontaneous vertebral fractures has shown a normal distribution. Thus, patients categorized as having high bone turnover are simply those who are on one end of this distribution. There is an equal number of women who could be categorized as having low bone turnover. There have been no studies to show that accelerated trabecular bone loss is the cause of postmenopausal osteoporosis. Furthermore, bone density of the proximal femur in women with Type I osteoporosis is as low as the bone density of the femur in individuals with Type II osteoporosis. It is likely that the fractures in elderly individuals are due to osteopenia, reduced bone quality and their increased propensity to fall. Older individuals may also tend to fall on their side (producing hip fracture) and have less musculature either to break or to reduce the impact of a fall.

Secondary osteoporosis

In 20% of women and 40% of men presenting with vertebral fractures a secondary cause of osteoporosis can be identified. The most common are early menopause (usually oophorectomy) in women, hypogonadism in men (occasionally hypopituitary (**176**), but usually hypergonadotrophic) (**177**), subtotal gastrectomy, chronic obstructive pulmonary disease, prior immobilization, and pharmacologic doses of glucocorticoid or thyroid hormones. The most commonly missed diagnoses are multiple myeloma and osteoporosis associated with alcoholism and disseminated carcinoma.

Since cancellous and endosteal surfaces are in contact with the marrow, disorders involving the bone marrow can change remodelling and lead to loss of cancellous and endocortical bone, with subsequent cortical thinning and expansion of the marrow cavity.

Multiple myeloma (**178, 179**) and macroglobulinaemia can be associated with bone disease. Usually there are multiple osteolytic lesions that may not show up on a bone scan. As a result of the number of bone resorbing cytokines produced it is not surprising that 1–2% of patients who present with generalized osteoporosis may have a plasma cell dyscrasia. In the elderly this must be differentiated from a benign monoclonal gammopathy, frequently requiring bone marrow examination.

176

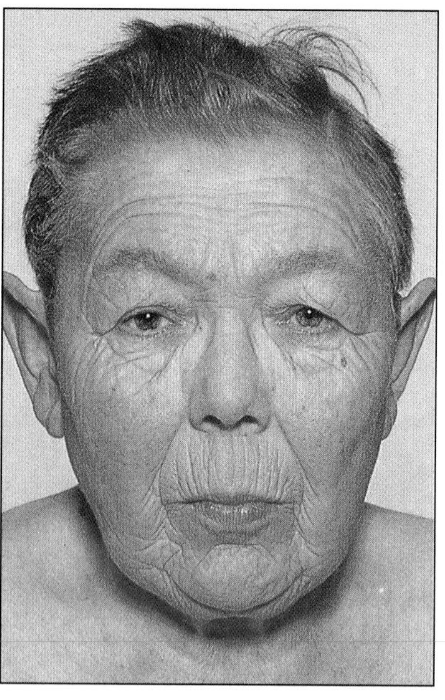

176 Hypopituitary hypogonadism.

177

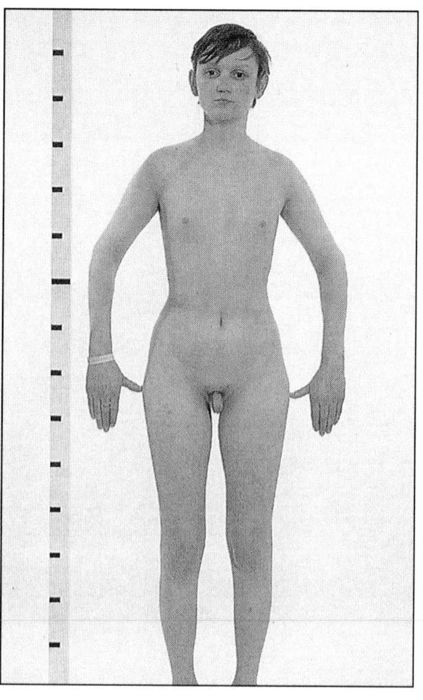

177 Hypergonadotrophic hypogonadism.

178

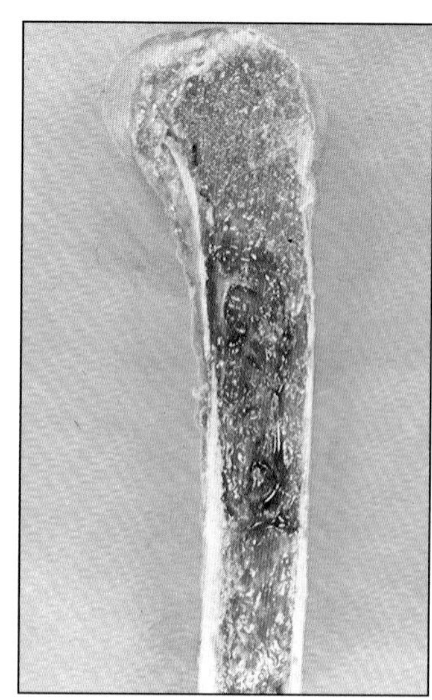

178 Multiple myeloma.

179

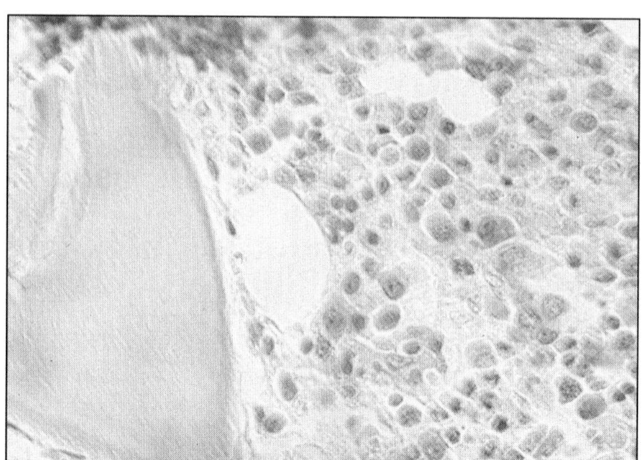

179 Multiple myeloma (magnification × 200).

180

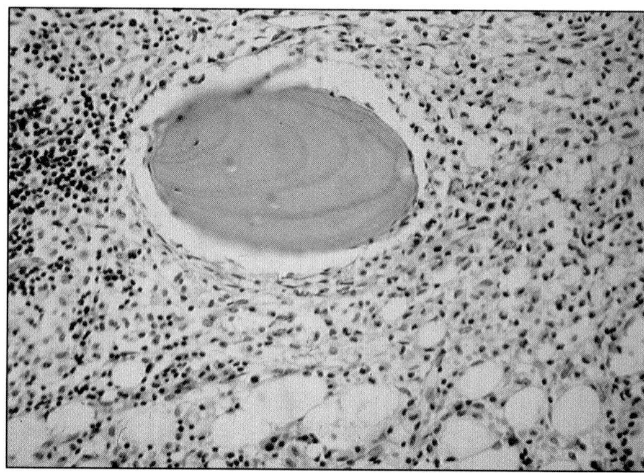

180 Mastocytosis (magnification × 100).

An abnormal proliferation of mast cells (mastocytosis) usually produces mixed sclerotic-porotic lesions and generalized osteoporosis is only rarely observed (**180**). Acute leukaemia, usually in adolescents, may produce diffuse osteoporosis of the spine. Transverse radiolucent bands at the metaphyses and focal osteolytic lesions are seen. Generalized osteopenia from lymphomatous involvement of the skeleton is rare. Hodgkin's disease in bone is shown in **181**. Sickle cell disease and thalassaemia minor can also result in osteopenia. In the former, the medullary cavity and intertrabecular spaces become widened with thinning of remaining trabeculae. Osteopenia is observed in the skull, mandible, and axial skeleton. There is widening of the diploic spaces and a coarse granular appearance to the vault with sparing of the occiput. Step-like indentations of the central portion of the vertebral end plates produce the 'H' vertebrae. In thalassaemia minor the whole skull is osteopenic with expansion of the facial bones leading to typical deformity. There is osteoporosis of the ribs and clavicle, and underconstriction and flaring of the distal femoral metaphysis (Ehrhenmeyer flask deformity).

Gaucher's disease produces vertebral fracture, and bony expansion with cortical thinning in the femur (**182**). There may be mixed lytic and sclerotic lesions. This disorder is much less common than Niemann–Pick disease.

181

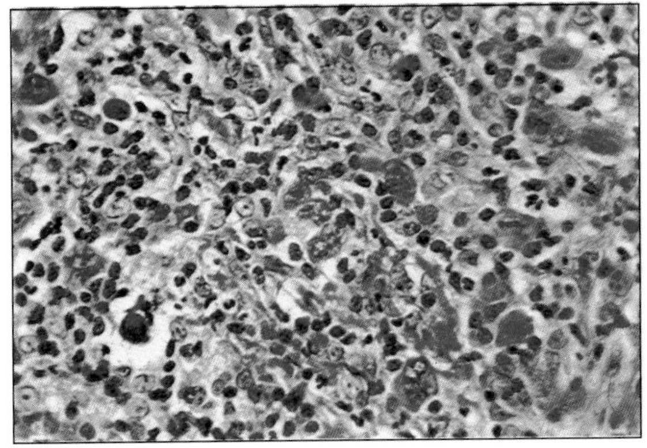

181 Hodgkin's disease (magnification × 100).

182

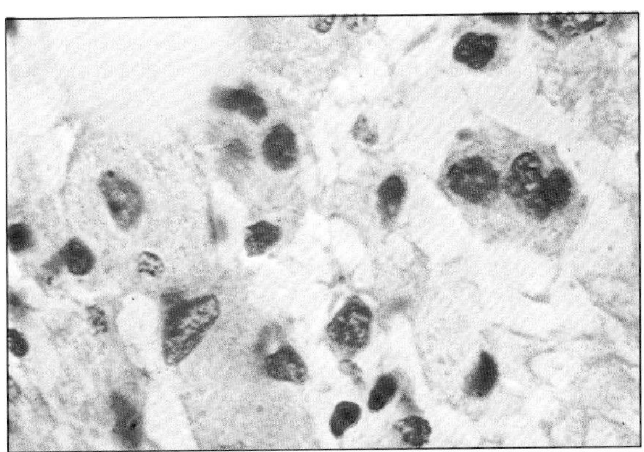

182 Gaucher's disease.

In Cushing's syndrome there is a decrease in calcium absorption with subsequent increased parathyroid hormone secretion, hypercalciuria, and increased activity of osteoclasts (**183**). Occasionally, a patient with Cushing's syndrome may present with osteoporotic fractures and not have all the physical signs of hypercortisolism. Of course, the use of glucocorticoid therapy is a much more common cause of osteoporosis than a spontaneous Cushing's disease.

Primary hyperparathyroidism has been diagnosed with increased frequency and it has recently been re-emphasized that osteitis fibrosa (**184**) may present clinically as the vertebral crush fracture syndrome. Normally, this is easily diagnosed by the presence of hypercalcaemia, but in patients with vitamin D deficiency or renal insufficiency hypercalcaemia may not be prominent.

183

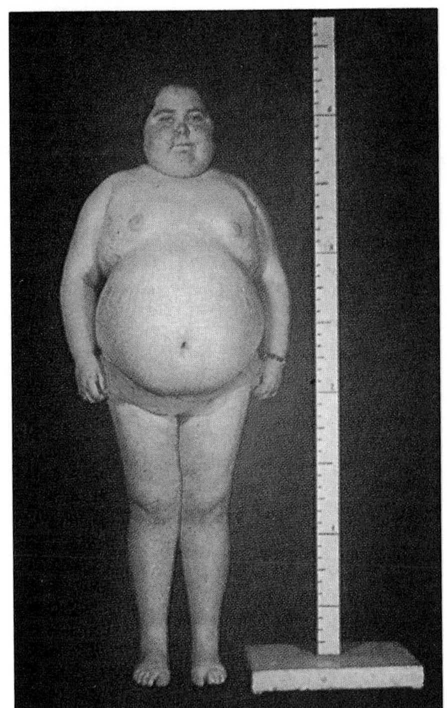

183 A patient with Cushing's syndrome.

184

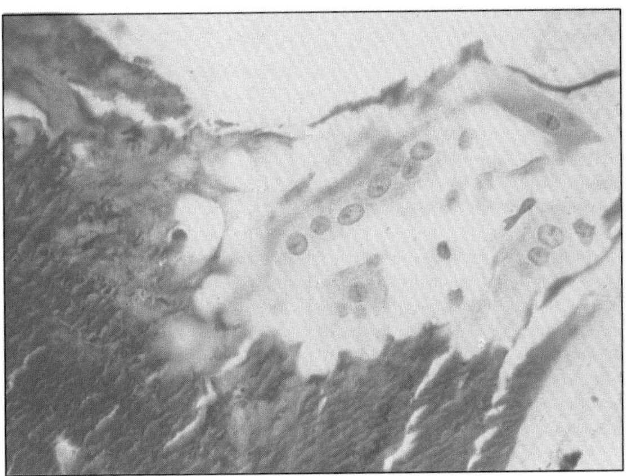

184 Osteitis fibrosa.

Hyperthyroidism (**185**) also produces a high bone turnover and can produce osteopenia of appendicular and axial bone. Occasionally, this is associated with fractures. A past history of hyperthyroidism should be elicited in risk assessment of women for osteoporosis. Excess thyroid hormone secretion produces increased bone resorption, decreased calcium absorption and hypercalciuria. Diabetes mellitus (Type I) has been associated with osteopenia. However, fracture studies have not revealed an increased incidence. The abnormal findings in Type I diabetes are: increased urinary excretion of calcium; decreased ionized calcium; normal to low blood levels of parathyroid hormone and 1,25-dihydroxyvitamin D; and a decreased bone formation rate. While the clinical significance of osteopenia in Type I diabetes remains controversial, it has been shown that there is no osteopenia in Type II diabetes.

A similar situation exists in patients with rheumatoid arthritis where osteopenia has been documented; however, the risk of fractures in patients who have not had drug therapy that produces osteopenia is unclear. Osteoporosis in rheumatoid arthritis starts with juxtarticular bone loss and eventually a generalized loss of bone density occurs. The osteopenia may result from decreased physical activity, but it has also been postulated that it is due to increased prostaglandins, cytokines and mast cell accumulation.

Acromegaly has been thought to be associated with osteoporosis (**186**). The metabolic bone disorder in acromegaly appears to reflect the re-emergence of the pattern of bone growth in a skeleton with fused epiphyses. There is an increase in periosteal apposition with increased turnover in trabecular bone. Studies of X-rays in acromegalic patients suggest that there is no increase in risk of fracture except when acromegaly is accompanied by hypogonadism. Growth hormone deficient children who have been treated until adulthood with growth hormone have osteopenia (**187**).

185

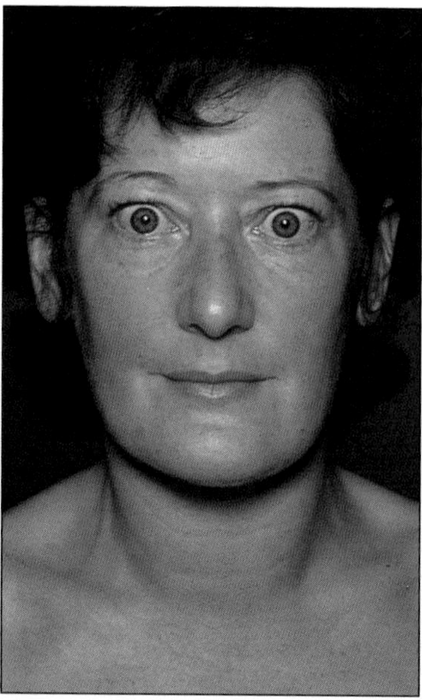

185 A patient with hyperthyroidism.

186

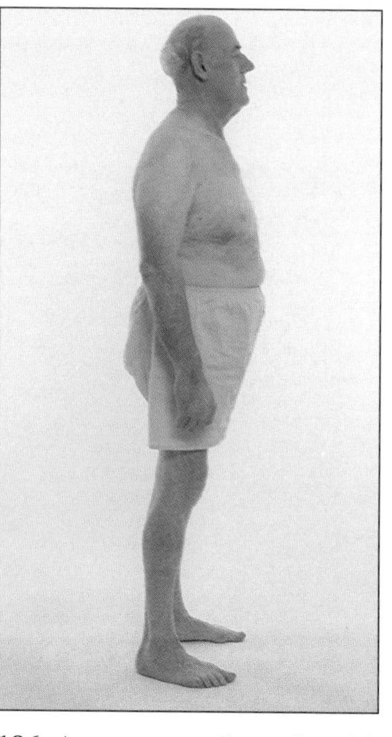

186 An acromegalic male with hypopituitarism.

187

187 A child with growth hormone deficiency.

Gastrointestinal disorders such as gastrectomy, hepatobiliary disease, intestinal surgery, as well as celiac disease (**188**), can result in malabsorption of calcium and osteopenia. There is a transient regional osteoporotic syndrome as well as the rare occurrence of osteoporosis in association with pregnancy and lactation (**189**). Regional osteoporosis is often an incidental finding that may be associated with limbs that have been immobilized for more than one month but may occur with the reflex dystrophy syndrome.

Fibrogenesis imperfectum osseous is a rare disease with generalized osteopenia and also a coarse and dense appearance of trabecular bone. In addition, osteogenesis imperfecta (**190, 191**) may present in later life with vertebral fractures. It is a heritable disorder which has been divided into four major types *(Table 23)*. The

188

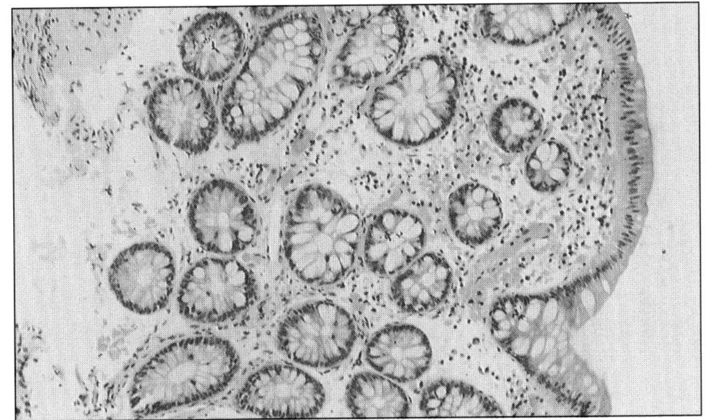

188 Celiac disease (magnification × 100).

189

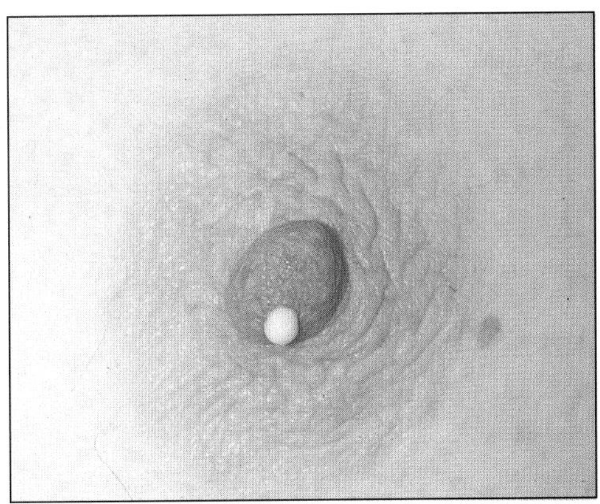

189 Osteoporosis can occasionally occur as a result of breast feeding.

disorder results from an abnormality of the synthesis or structure of the most abundant form of collage found in matrix, Type I collagen. Osteogenesis imperfecta is associated with recurrent fracture and skeletal deformity but may also be related to abnormal dentinogenesis, joint hypermobility, excessive diaphoresis, hearing loss, and blue sclera (**192–196**). There may be evidence of osteopenia, prior to puberty, in patients with Turner's syndrome; this suggests that it is not only the hypogonadism which produces osteopenia (**197**). Sarcoidosis, haemochromatosis, prolonged parenteral nutrition, and any state that produces severe malnutrition (**198**) may be associated with osteoporosis.

190

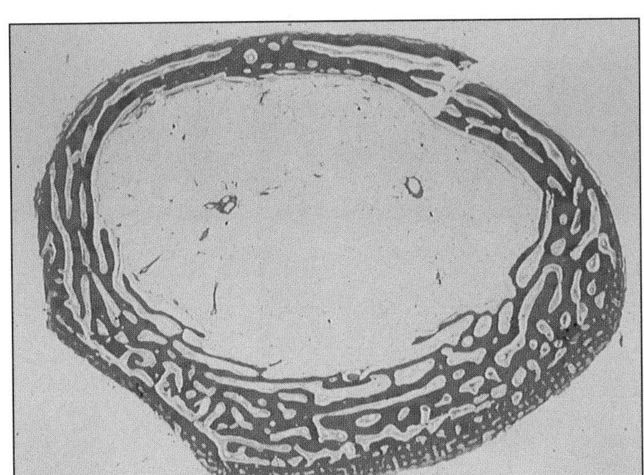

191

190, 191 Osteogenesis imperfecta at a low magnification (**190**) and at a high magnification (**191**).

Table 23. Types of osteogenesis imperfecta.

Type	*Clinical features*	*Inheritance*
I	Normal stature, little or no deformity, blue scleras, hearing loss (50%); dentinogenesis imperfecta rare	Autosomal dominant
II	Lethal in the perinatal period, minimal calvarial mineralization, beaded ribs, compressed femurs, platyspondylia, marked long bone deformity	Autosomal dominant (rarely recessive)
III	Progressively deforming bones with deformity at birth; scleras variable in hue, often lighten with age; dentinogenesis imperfecta, hearing loss, stature very short	Autosomal recessive Autosomal dominant
IV	Normal scleras, mild to moderate bone deformity and variable short stature, dentinogenesis imperfecta, hearing loss in some	Autosomal dominant

192

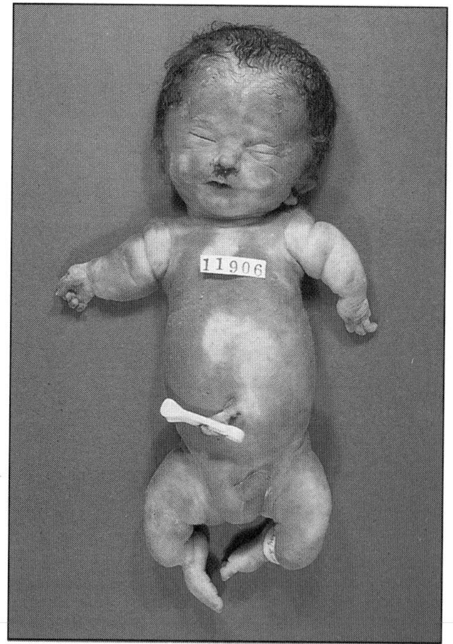

193

192 Osteogenesis imperfecta, Type II.

193 X-ray of the baby shown in **192**.

194

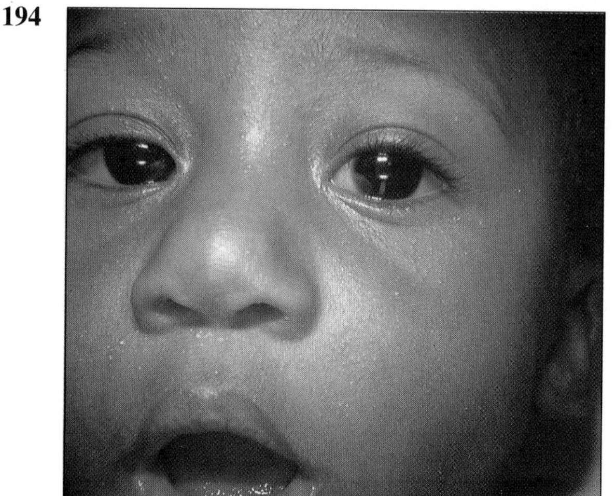
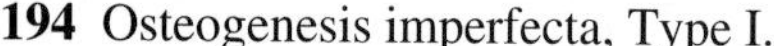

194 Osteogenesis imperfecta, Type I.

195

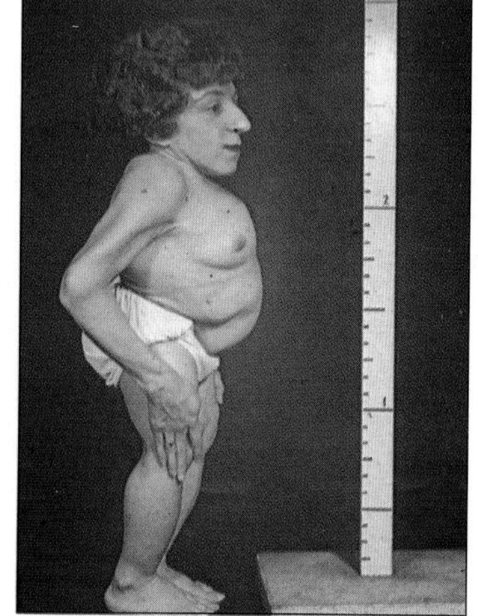

195 Osteogenesis imperfecta, Type III.

196

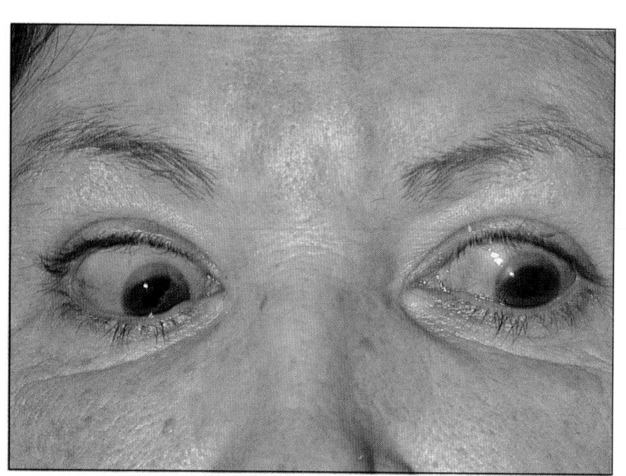

196 Osteogenesis imperfecta with blue sclera.

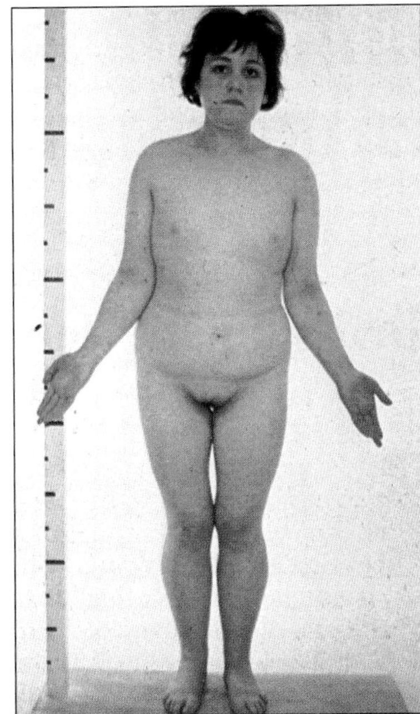

197 A patient with Turner's syndrome.

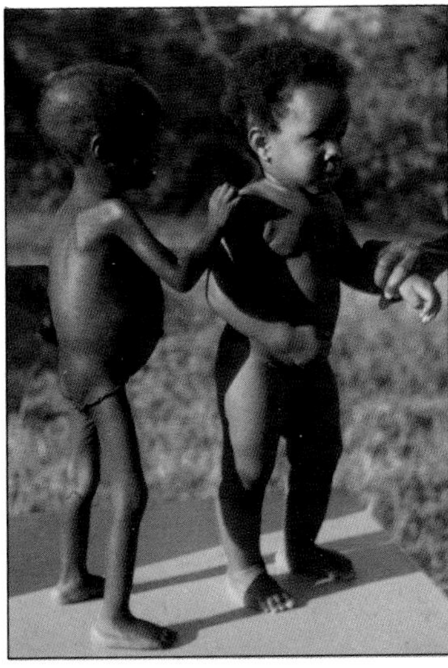

198 Marasmus in a child is associated with osteoporosis.

The osteopenia associated with total parenteral nutrition is high turnover, followed by osteomalacia and associated with peri-articular bone pain. This may be an example of toxins regulating bone turnover because of the presence of aluminum in the case of hydroxylate. A similar picture may develop in patients undergoing haemodialysis. Scurvy may be responsible for osteoporosis in infancy with a ground glass appearance inradiographs. Disuse osteoporosis most often accompanies neurologic disorders such as polio, stroke, and spinal cord injury. Any cause of secondary hyperparathyroidism, including renal hypercalciuria, malabsorption syndromes, and chronic renal insufficiency may result in osteopenia.

Drug therapy

Glucocorticoid therapy is one of the most common causes of drug-induced osteoporosis. High-dose glucocorticoids frequently produce this disorder. Whereas premenopausal women do not seem to be affected by low-dose prednisone therapy (i.e. less than 7.5mg per day), postmenopausal women on the same dose lose bone rapidly. There is speculation that the increased sensitivity of postmenopausal women to glucocorticoids may be due to the menopausal decrease in ovarian androgen production. Alternate-day steroid day therapy does not reduce the effect of steroids on calcium metabolism. Thyroid replacement therapy has been associated with osteopenia. The cause of replacement therapy causing osteopenia is unknown. However, the development of the ultrasensitive assay for thyroid stimulating hormone has shown that the majority of patients who had previously been on thyroxine replacement therapy were overdosed. Average replacement therapies of L-thyroxine with the newer assays has led to a reduction in average doses from 0.15mg per day to less than 0.1mg per day. It is hoped that with the use of the ultrasensitive TSH assay the osteopenia induced by thyroxine replacement therapy will no longer occur.

Anti-convulsant therapy is also associated with osteoporosis and osteomalacia. The mechanism of action is probably related to the induction of hepatic microsomal enzyme activity and subsequent alteration of vitamin D metabolism. Long-term heparin use produces osteopenia. Lithium therapy results in an increase in parathyroid hormone secretion and may lead to hypercalcaemia and osteopenia. The effect of cytotoxic agents on mineralized tissue results in bone loss. The use of GnRH or LHRH antagonists or agonist treatment is also associated with bone loss. Some studies have implicated theophylline, phenothiazine derivatives

199

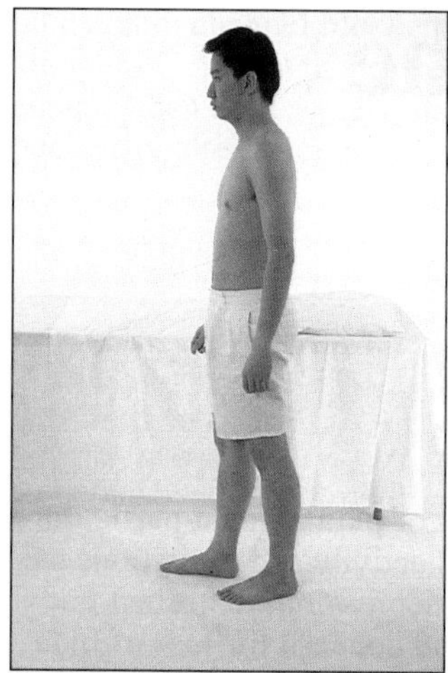

199 Patient walking on the balls of his feet and heels.

200

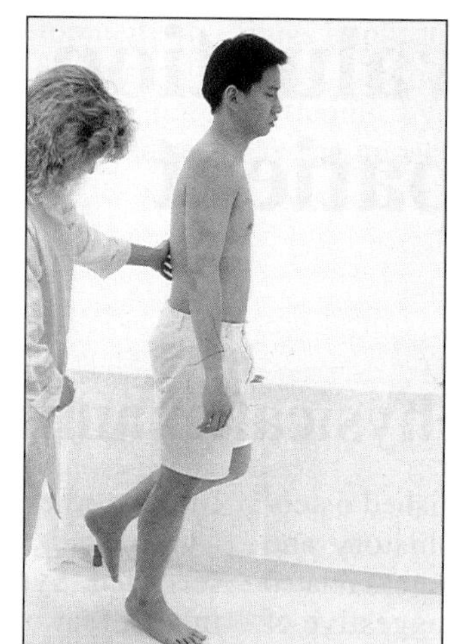

200 The Trendellenberg test.

201

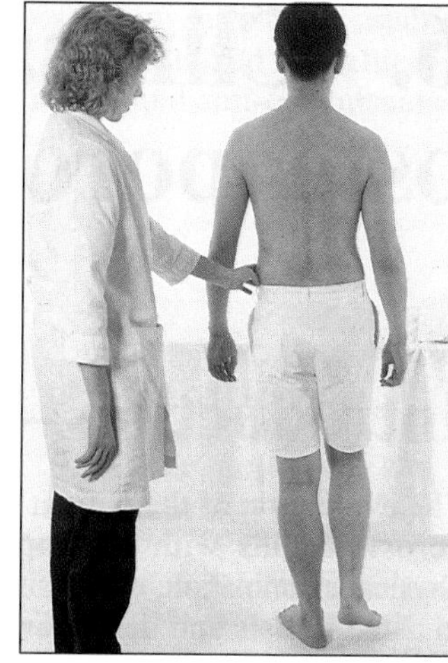

201 Examination of the posterior superior iliac spines.

202

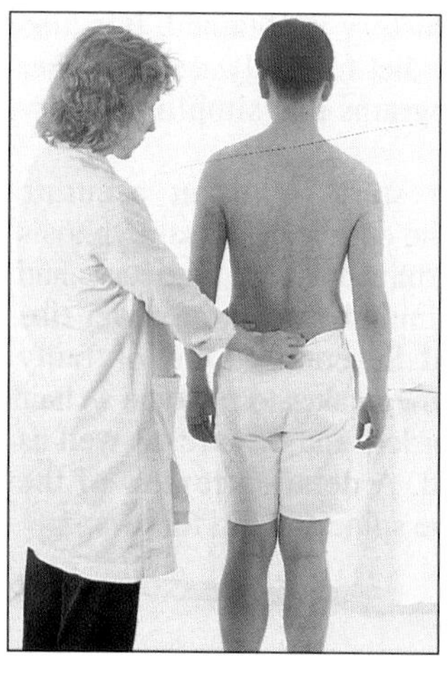

202 Examination of the skin folds.

203

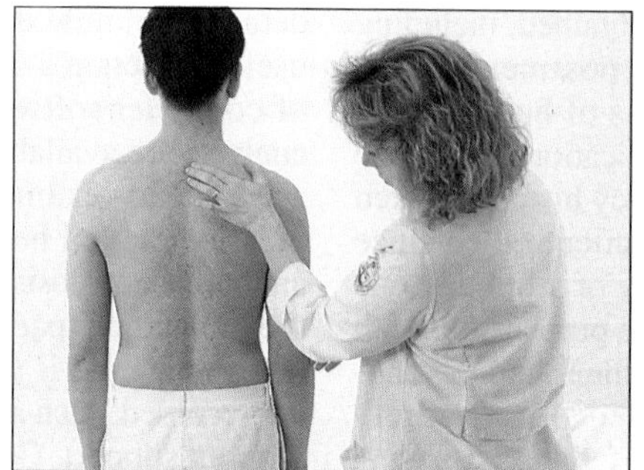

203 The performance of palpation.

204

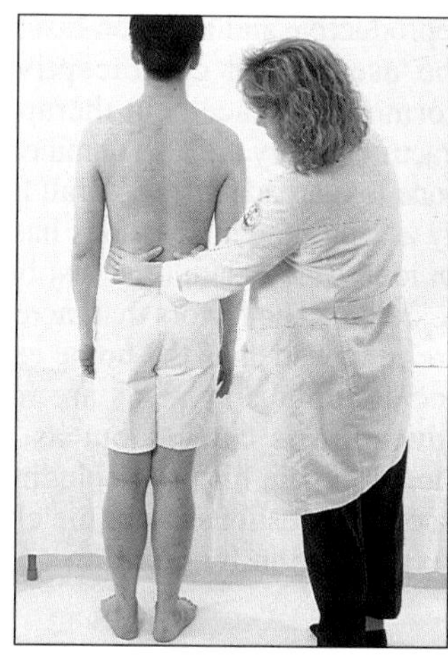

204 Examination to determine the space between the lower ribs and pelvic brim.

205

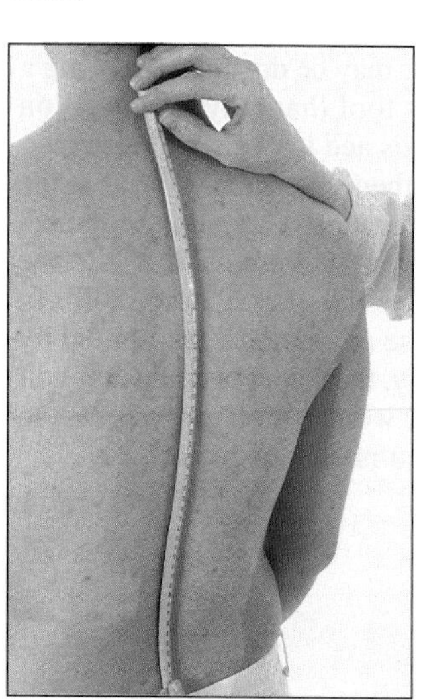

206

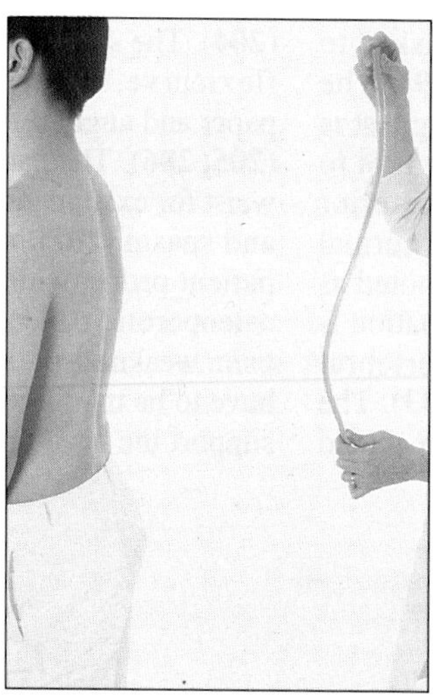

205, 206 The measurement of the angles of kyphosis and lordosis using a flexicurve.

207

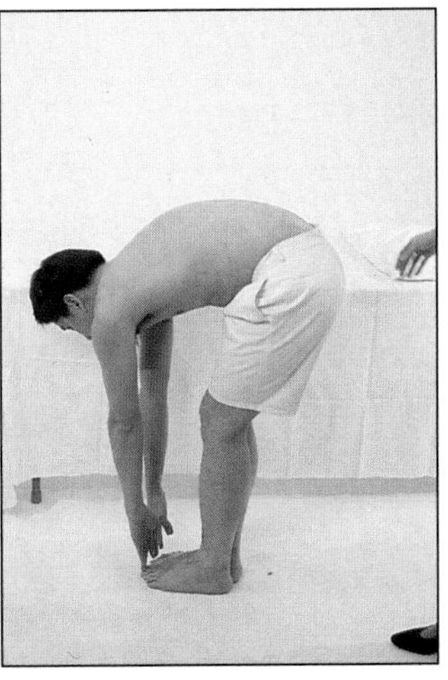

207 Examination to determine limitation of motion, tenderness and spasm.

208

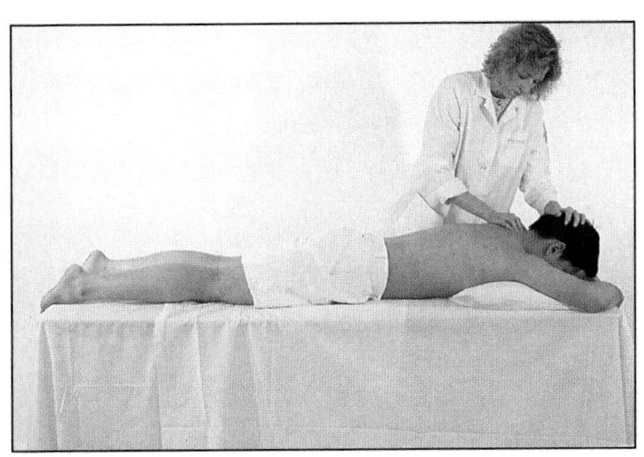

208 The same examination as in **207**, but with the patient in the prone position.

Manoeuvres to help determine the aetiology of pain include the femoral stretch test in which the hip is passively extended (**209**) , straight leg raising (**210**), and Luseck's manoeuvre (passive dorsiflexion of the foot (**211**). Flexion of the knee (**212**) may relieve either sciatic or hamstring pain but may also reproduce pain with mechanical origin in the lumbosacral spine.

209

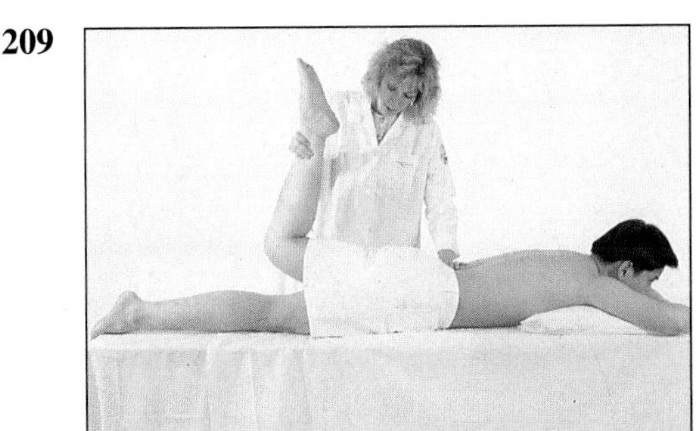

209 Femoral stretch test.

210

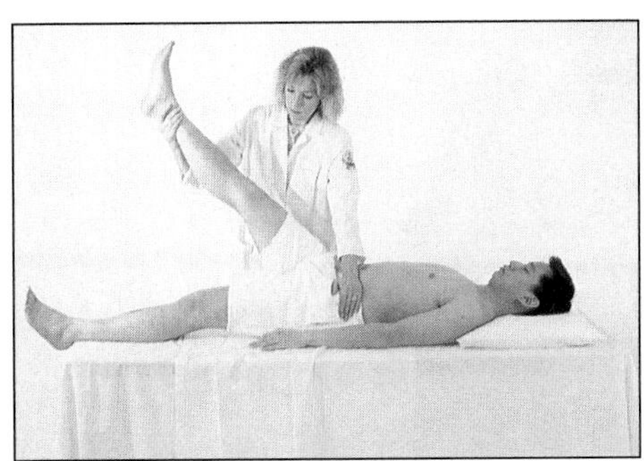

210 Straight leg raising.

211

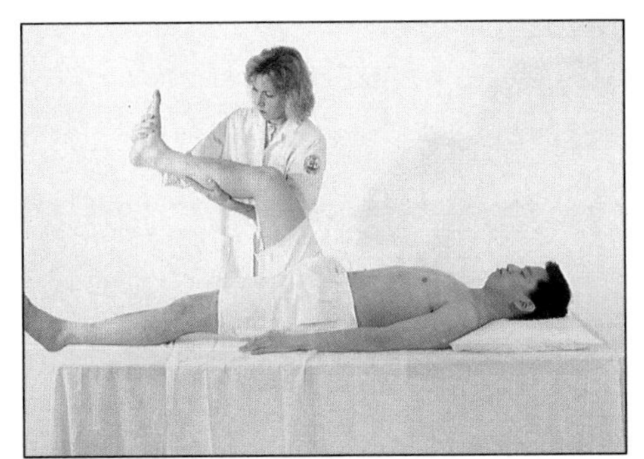

211 Luseck's manoeuvre.

212

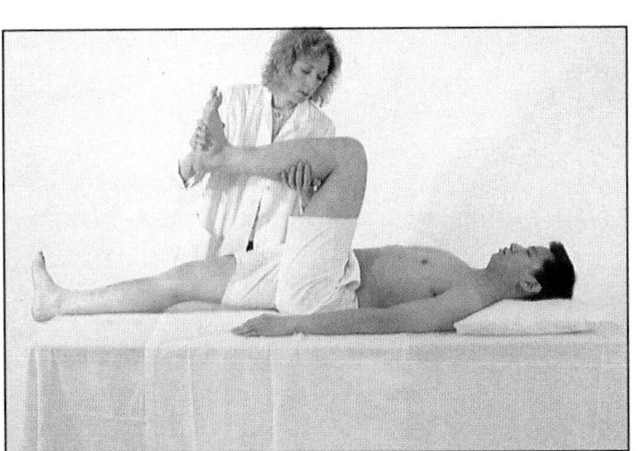

212 Knee flexion.

Examination of the extremities must demonstrate mobility, strength, and neurologic function and sources of pain. **213–220** show various manoeuvres.

213

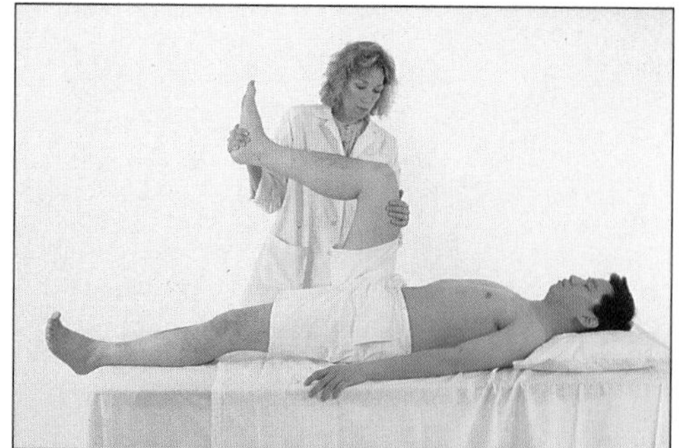

213 Flexion of the hip to 90°.

214

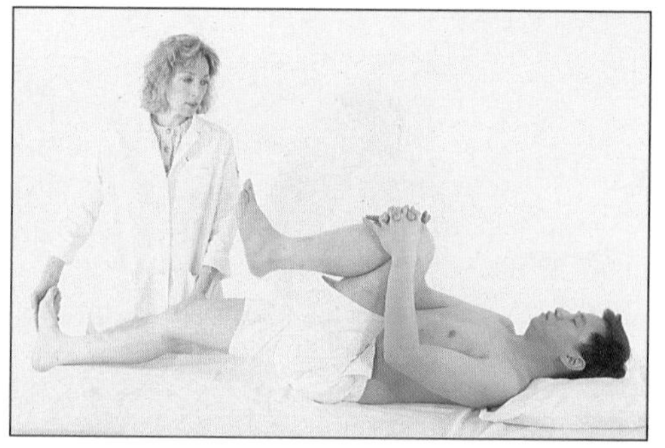

214 The Thomas test: locking one hip and extending the opposite hip to test for flexion contracture.

215

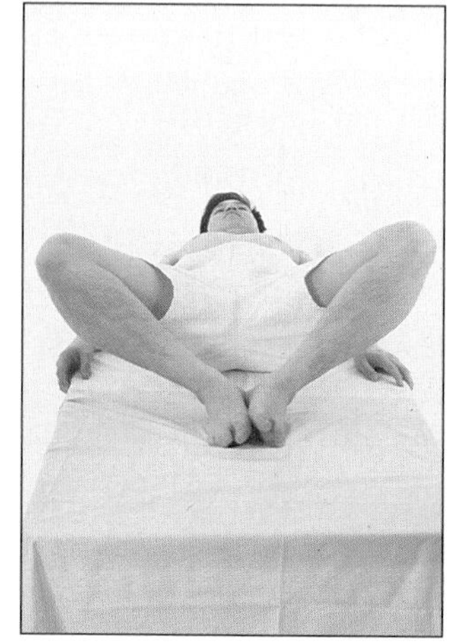

215 Adduction in a 45° flexion.

216

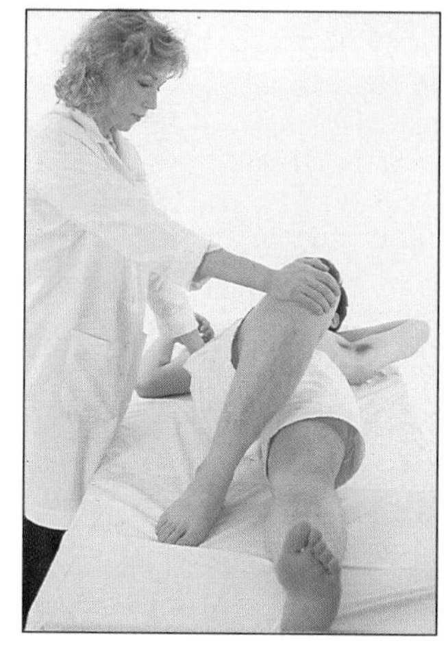

216 In flexion.

217

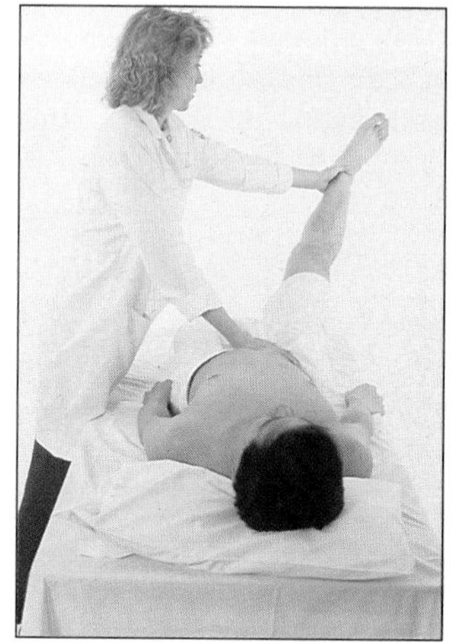

217 In extension.

218

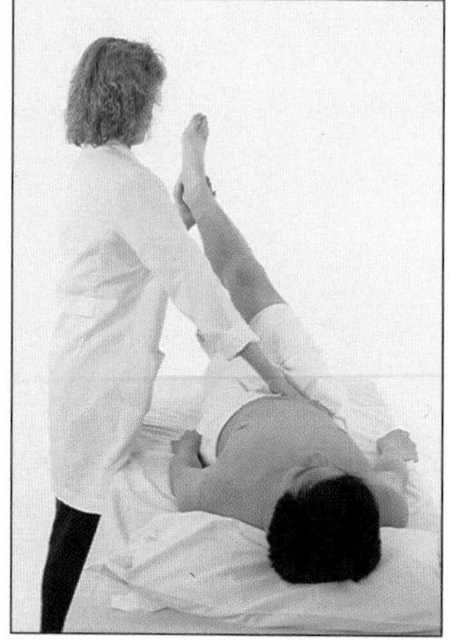

218 Adduction in extension.

219

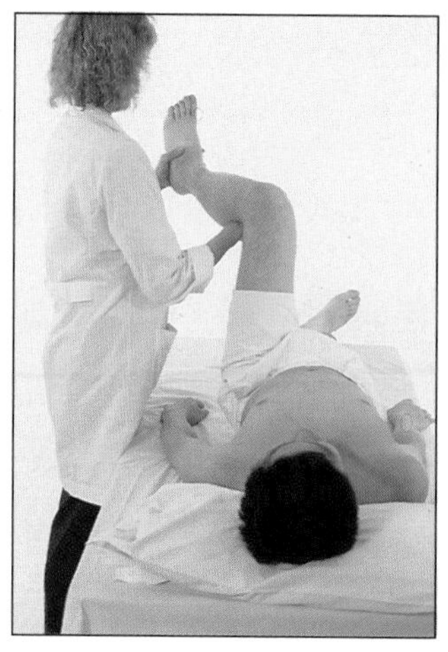

219 External rotation.

220

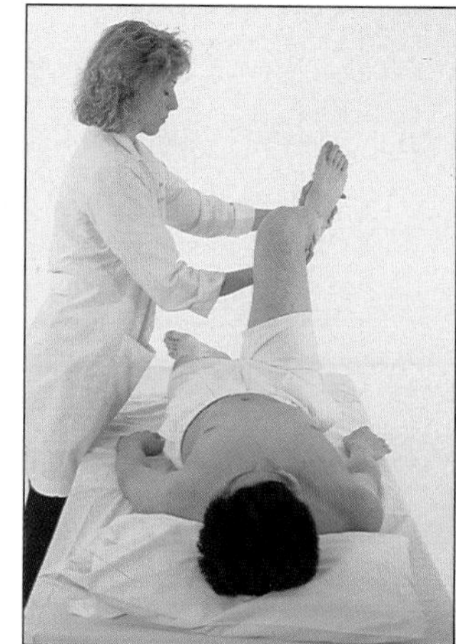

220 Internal rotation.

The hip extensors are tested with the patient prone and the knee flexed to 90° (**221**) in external and internal rotation. A variety of manoeuvres are carried out to test for muscle strength (**222, 223**). A comprehensive stepwise test of muscle strength and neurologic function is conducted. Leg length is measured from the anterior iliac spine to the middle of the medial malleus (**224**).

221

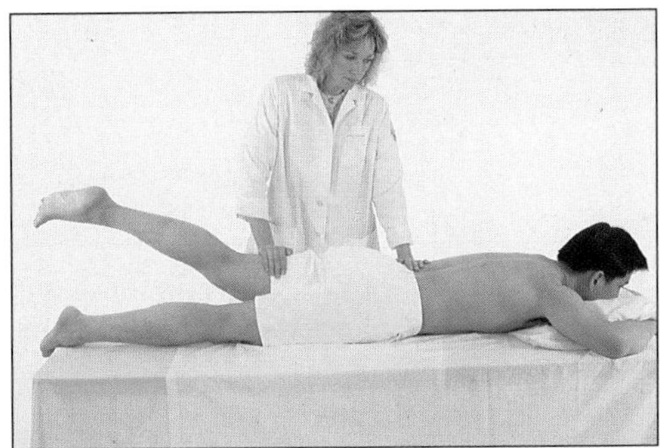

221 Hip extensors.

222

222 The deep knee bend.

223

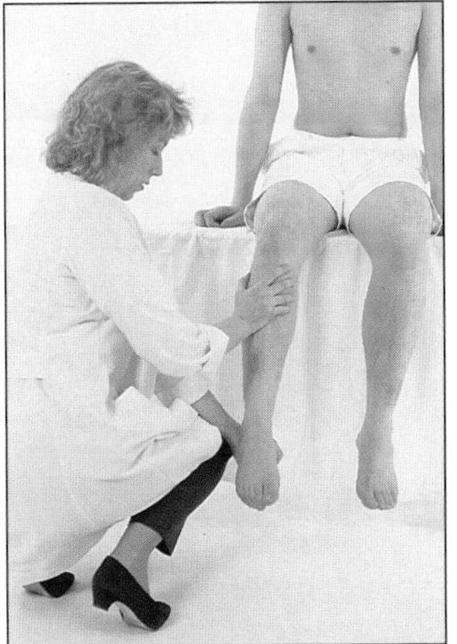

223 A test for the strength of the hamstrings.

224

224 Measuring the leg length of a patient.

Examination of the spine of a woman with multiple vertebral compression fractures is demonstrated in **225–231**.

225

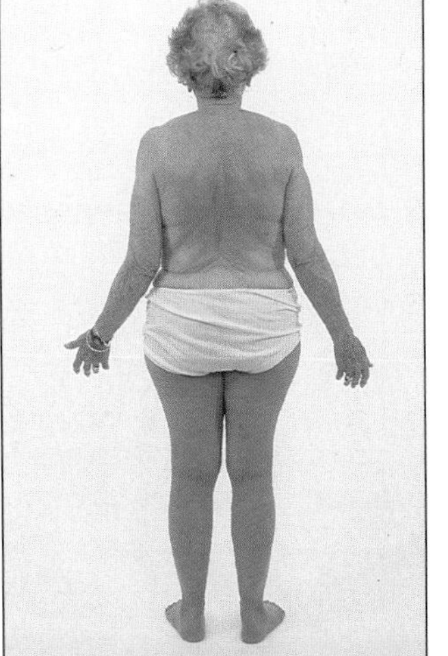

225 The patient shows kyphosis with a suggestion of shortening of the thoracic spine when examined from behind.

226

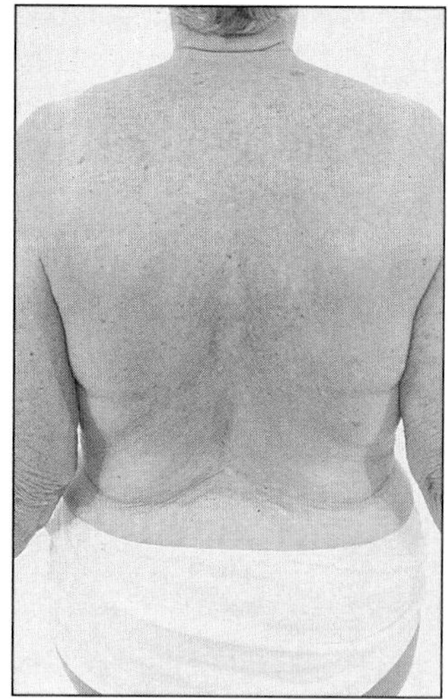

227

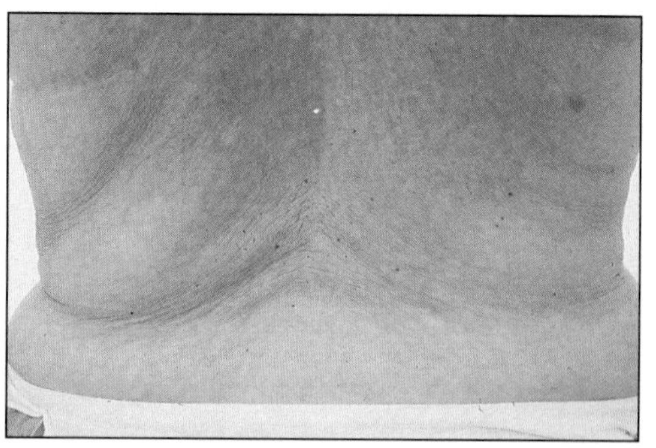

226, 227 The skin folds shown in these two figures are further evidence of shortening of the spine.

228

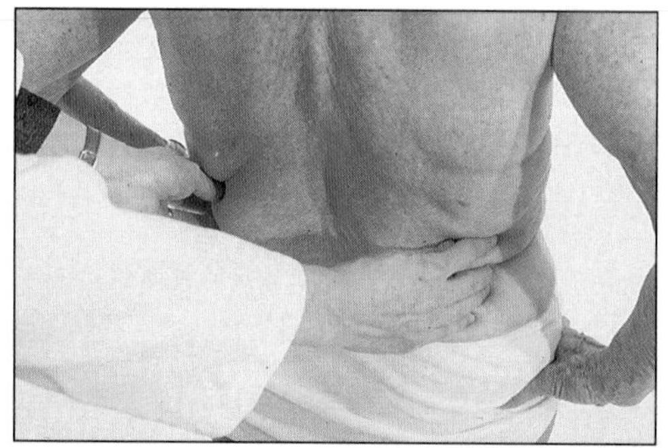

228 Palpation demonstrates the virtual absence of space between the lower rib cage and the pelvic brim.

229

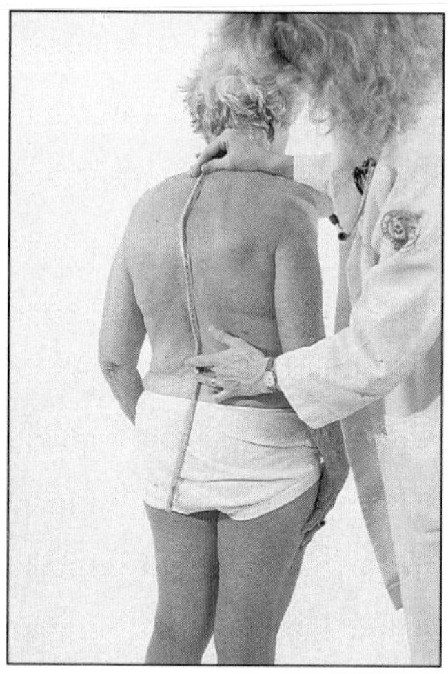

229 The flexicurve is traced on paper to record improvement in kyphosis with physical therapy.

230

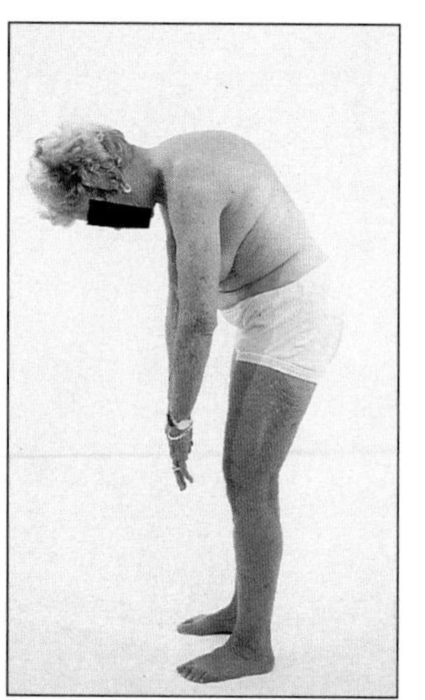

230 Kyphosis is more apparent in the lateral view as shown here; limitation of motion is also apparent.

231

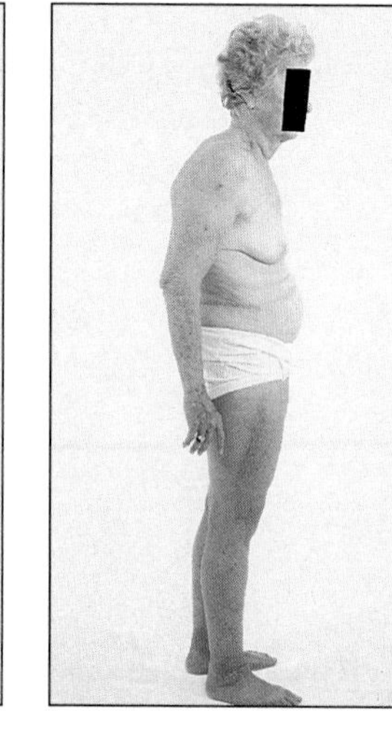

231 With the patient standing sideways, the following can be noted: kyphosis with loss of normal lordosis; the arms appear disproportionately longer than the trunk (due to vertebral compression); and the proturberance of the abdomen (because there is no room for abdominal contents).

Laboratory and radiographic examination

The object of the laboratory examination is to find secondary causes of osteopenia. Routine tests, including a complete blood count urinalysis, multi-channel chemistry profile, free thyroxine, ultrasensitive TSH and serum protein electrophoresis, are carried out. If persistent pain or anaemia suggest myeloma, a serum and urine immunoelectrophoresis is performed. A bone marrow test may also be performed to exclude myeloma or to look for metastatic disease. If weight loss or stool characteristics indicate malabsorption, then serum 25-hydroxyvitamin D, parathyroid hormone, and 24-hour urine analyses for calcium are performed (plus serum carotene and faecal fat). The 24-hour urine analysis for calcium is also undertaken if there is a family or personal history of kidney stones and may be performed in all patients as a guide to how much calcium is being absorbed. If there is evidence of an endocrinopathy or other secondary osteoporoses, appropriate specialized tests will be ordered.

Biochemical markers of bone turnover may be useful in assessing whether the patient is undergoing high bone turnover as well as in following response to treatment. Bone formation markers include total and skeletal-specific alkaline phosphatase, serum osteocalcin, and serum Type I procollagen peptides. Serum osteocalcin is the most useful measure of osteoblast activity. Fasting urinary calcium and hydroxyproline have been used for years as markers of bone resorption. Recently developed markers of bone resorption include pyridinoline cross-links of collagen and plasma tartrate resistant acid phosphatase (TRAP); currently, however, pyridinoline cross-link assays (as a measure of osteoblastic activity) have shown to be more successful. Since a single low bone density may have resulted from a low peak bone mass or current rapid bone loss, it is hoped that the levels of markers of bone turnover can distinguish these situations and assist in clinical decision making regarding appropriate therapy.

An X-ray of the thoracic and lumbosacral spine is reviewed and abnormalities recorded. If pain is persistent or generalized, and is present only on standing or radiates down the leg, computed tomography or magnetic imaging may be performed. It must always be remembered that it cannot be assumed that osteoporosis is the cause of pain, even when there is a classic vertebral compression fracture. If there is a history or suspicion of a neoplasm a bone scan may be ordered. The baseline bone density of the spine and/or femur is measured. If there is scoliosis, abnormal aortic calcification or compression fractures in the area to be scanned, the femur is a preferable site to scan because its measurement is not confounded by these possible sources of error. The measurement of the bone mineral density of the femoral neck is as low as the spine measurement, even in women who present with vertebral fractures. Other alternatives are to measure total body bone mineral or bone mineral density of the radius.

The bone biopsy

Histomorphometric analysis of trabecular bone biopsies using fluorochromes to measure mineral apposition rate has provided a great deal of information concerning bone remodelling dynamics and is indicated in selected patients with osteopenia. Demeclocycline (150mg four times a day) or tetracycline (250mg four times a day) is given for 3 days; 2 weeks later it is administered for another 3 days, and then, 5 days later, the biopsy is performed. The distance between the two labels provides the mineral apposition rate.

The biopsy may be done as an outpatient procedure under local anaesthesia. A variety of trephines can be used, but they should have an inner diameter of 7.5–8.0mm; the operator should have an instrument with sharp teeth (**232**) and must apply gentle pressure. The

232

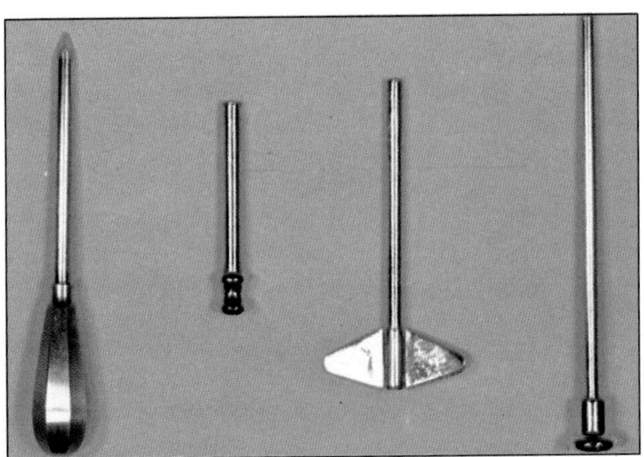

232 A selection of trephines.

specimen is placed in 70% ethanol and later imbedded in methyl methacrylate or another hard plastic and cut with an appropriate microtome (**233**). Unstained sections are used with epifluorescence to measure the distance between fluorescent bands, and a variety of stains can be used for light microscopy. A double tetracycline label in newly formed bone is seen in **234** and in a rim of osteoid with active osteoblasts in **235**. Lamellar osteoid, seen in osteomalacia, is shown in **236**. Osteocytes may be seen within the newly formed bone in **237**, and the ruffled border of an osteoclast is seen in **238**. A biopsy from an osteoporotic patient with high bone remodelling is shown in **239**. The basic measurements which are taken are trabecular bone volume (TV/BV), bone surface (BS), eroded surface (ES/BS), osteoid surface (OS/BS), mineralized surface (MS/BS), wall thickness (W.Th), osteoid thickness (O.Th), and mineral apposition rate (NAR). Measurements can be calculated using automated equipment (**240**).

233

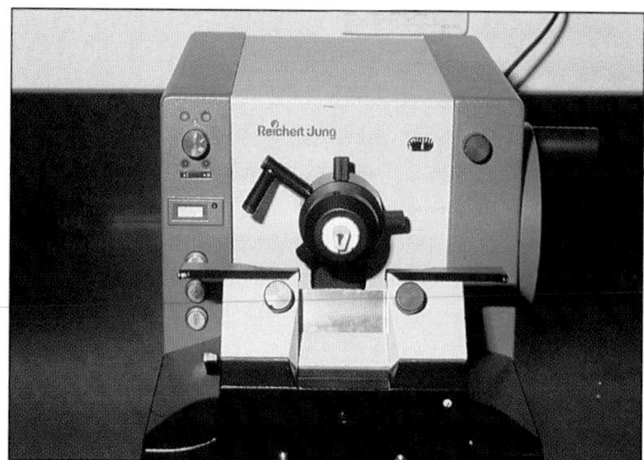

233 A microtome for sectioning undecalcified bone.

234

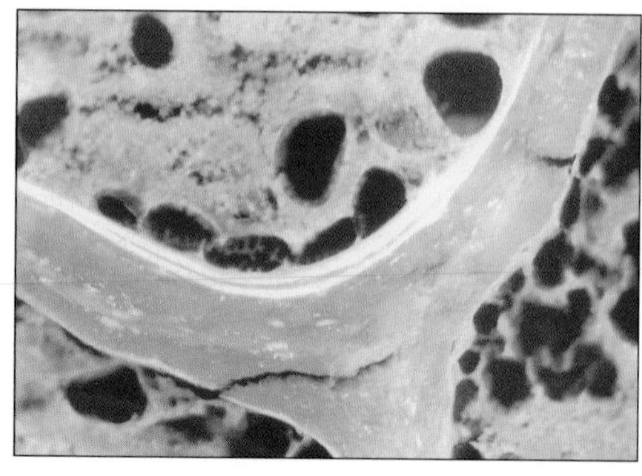

234 A double tetracycline label in newly formed bone.

235

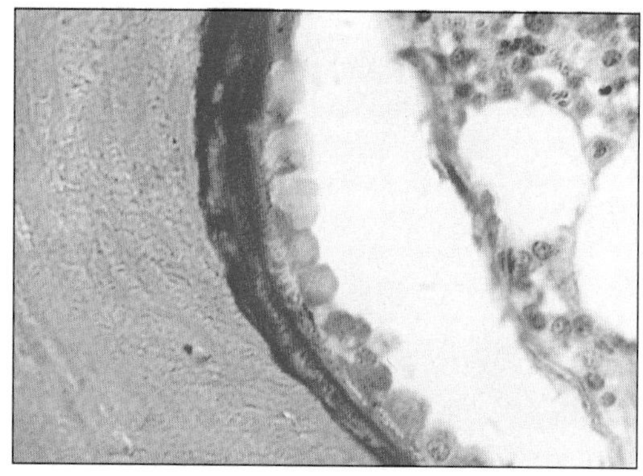

235 A double tetracycline label in a rim of osteoid with active osteoblasts.

236

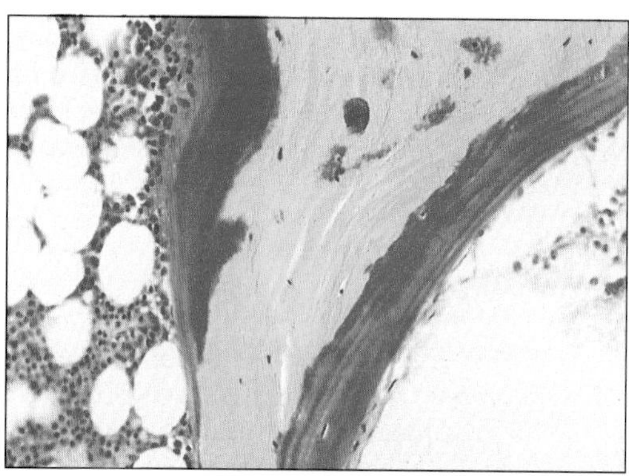

236 Lamellar osteoid.

237

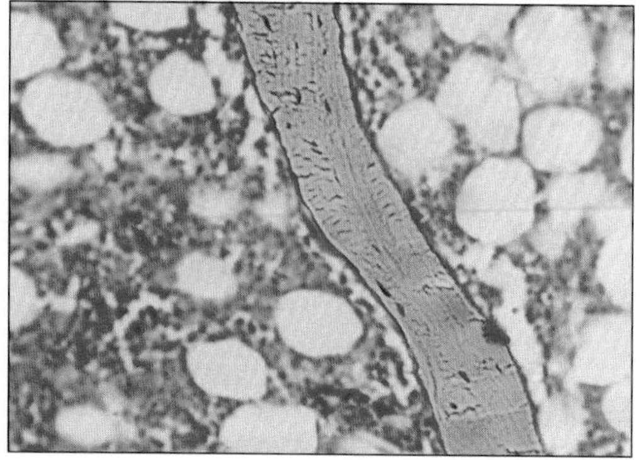

237 Osteocytes within the newly formed bone.

238

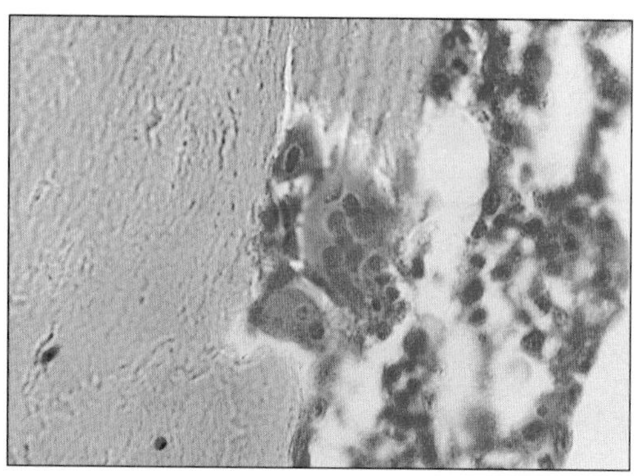

238 The ruffled border of an osteoclast.

239

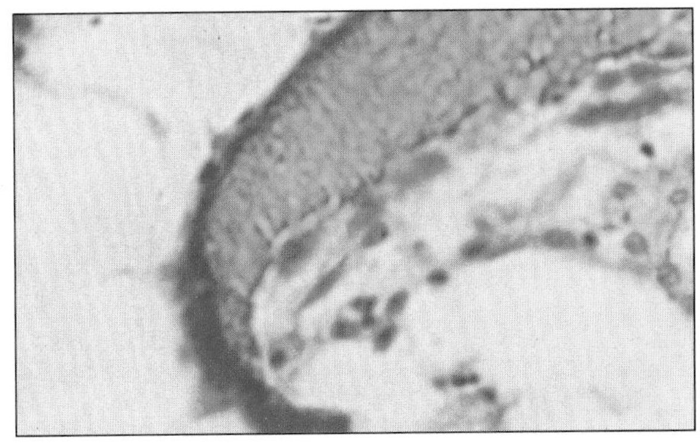

239 A biopsy from an osteoporotic patient with high bone remodelling.

240

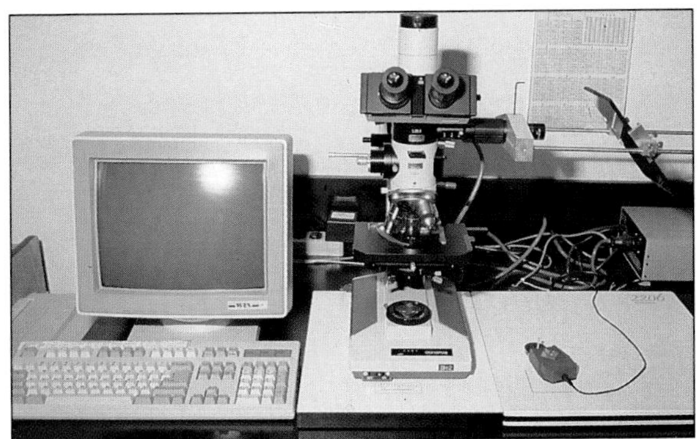

240 Automated equipment for measuring bone remodelling.

The major indications for bone biopsy are in metabolic bone disorders other than osteoporosis (**241–245**), e.g. vitamin D resistant rickets (**241**), renal osteodystrophy (**242, 243**), aluminum bone disease (**244**), nutritional rickets and osteomalacia (**245**), chronic gastrointestinal and liver disease, osteopenia with GI surgery, and anticonvulsant osteomalacia. Osteitis fibrosa cystica may be found (**246**).

241

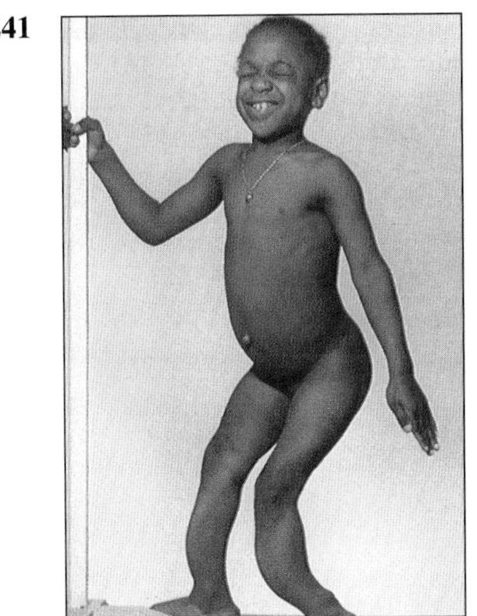

241 Vitamin D resistant rickets.

242

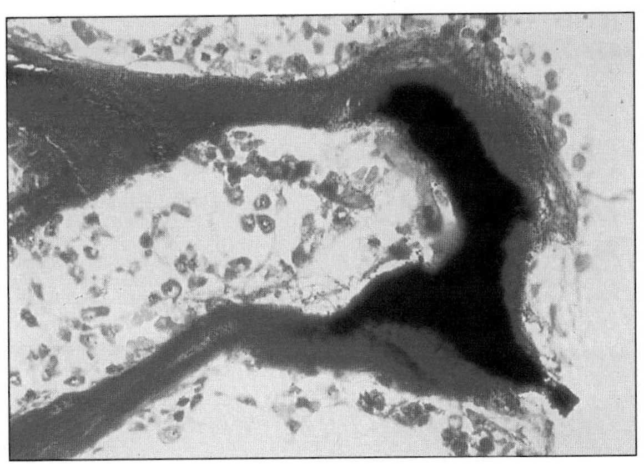

242 Renal osteodystrophy.

243

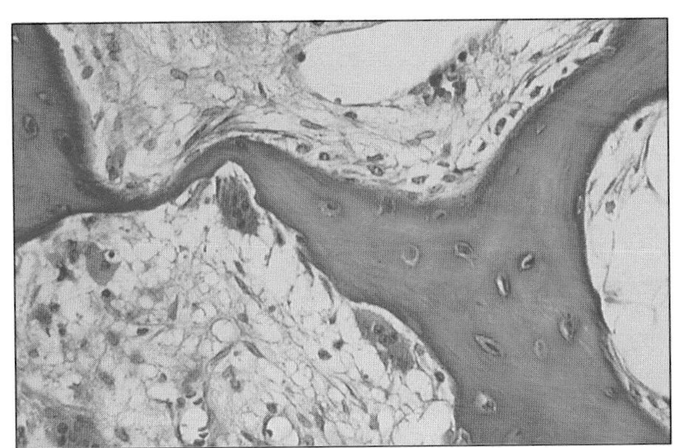

243 Renal osteitis.

244

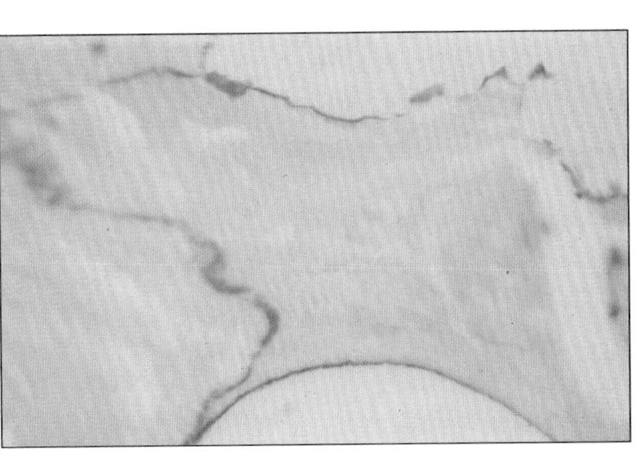

244 Aluminum bone disease.

245 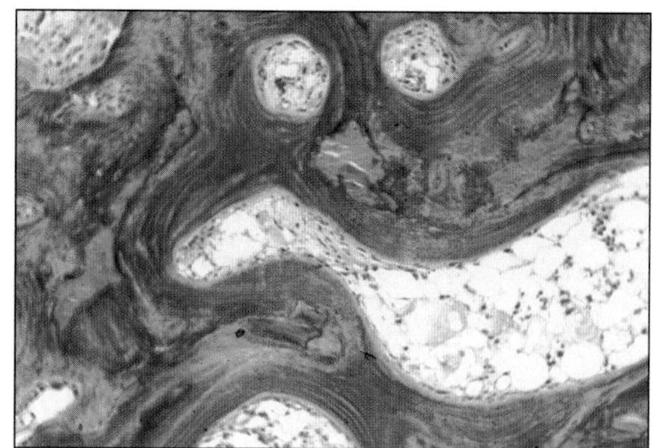

245 Nutritional osteomalacia (Goldner's stain × 150).

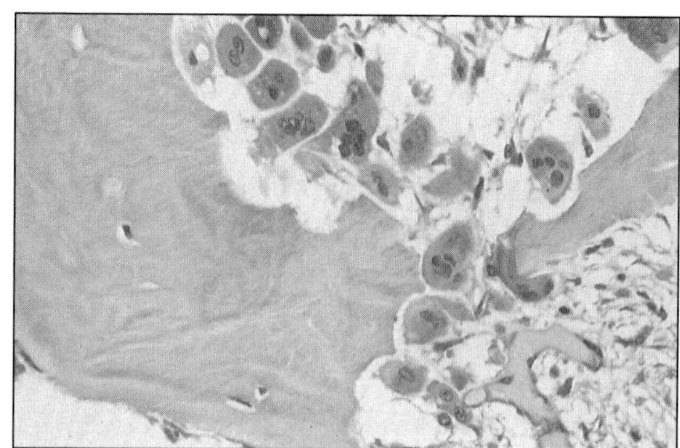 24

246 Osteitis fibrosa cystica.

247 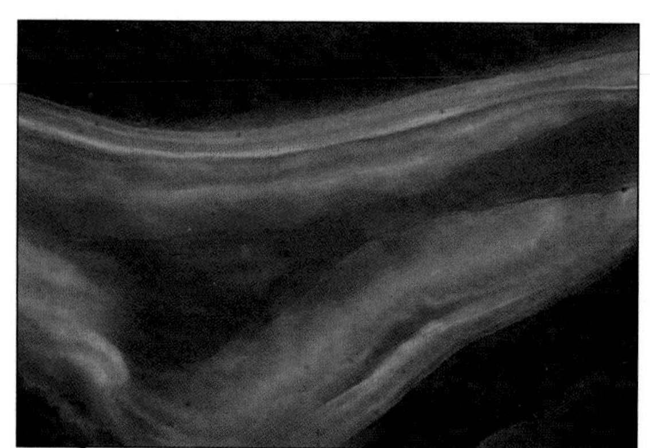

247 Multiple tetracycline labels (fluorescent light × 200).

The multiple tetracycline labels that may be seen in osteomalacia are shown in **247**. In a patient with classic osteoporosis it is usually unnecessary to do a bone biopsy. However, if there is any suspicion that another cause of osteopenia may be present, then the biopsy is indicated. Moreover, biopsy may be considered in atypical cases such as in a menstruating woman with no risk factors for osteoporosis.

7. Radiology in osteoporosis

Radiological diagnosis

Roentgenographs are useful in determining vertebral shape and in differentiating between the various causes of vertebral deformity as well as osteopenia. However, since osteoporosis can only be diagnosed by the elimination of other causes of osteopenia, conclusions from X-rays should only state that the findings are consistent with osteoporosis. The characteristic changes include the following:

- Generalized osteopenia.
- Thinning and accentuation of the cortex.
- Accentuation of primary trabeculae and loss of secondary trabeculae.
- Changes in vertebral shape (bio-concavity, wedge-shape, compression).
- Fracture of bones predisposed to osteoporosis (typically the spine, femur, wrist and rib).

Intracortical and trabecular bone resorption occur, in postmenopausal osteoporosis (and other high turnover conditions). Endosteal resorption predominates in Type II (involutional) osteoporosis, and subperiosteal resorption characterizes excess parathyroid hormone secretion. The loss of secondary trabeculae with the accentuation of primary trabeculae results in the striated appearance of the vertebral body. (In osteomalacia, the primary trabeculae appear indistinct.) Because of the loss of cancellous bone, the cortices of the vertebral body appear accentuated; they are referred to as the 'empty box' or 'picture framing' and there is angling of the end-plates. Unfortunately, the reliability of most of these findings is poor, due to such factors as artifacts from breathing, varied radiation exposure and positioning errors. Therefore, emphasis has been placed on vertebral shape.

As a result of the decreased density of the vertebral body, the intervertebral disc protrudes into the adjacent vertebral body, causing bending of the end-plates (bio-concavity). The thickness of the cortex is reduced. Protrusion of the disc material into the vertebral body (Schmorl's node) is of no diagnostic significance. Eventually, because of weakness of the vertebral structure and the anterior aspect of the vertebrae, compression fractures occur. **248–256** show various aspects of osteopenia.

248

248 Generalized osteopenia in the frontal and occipital regions in a 70-year-old woman with osteoporosis.

249

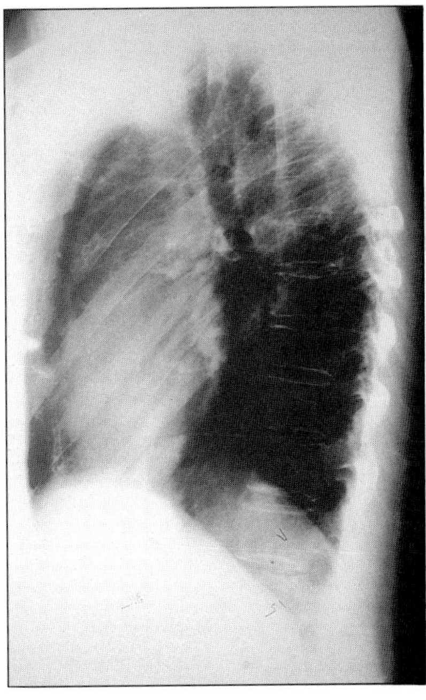

249 Generalized osteopenia of the spine in the woman seen in **248**.

250

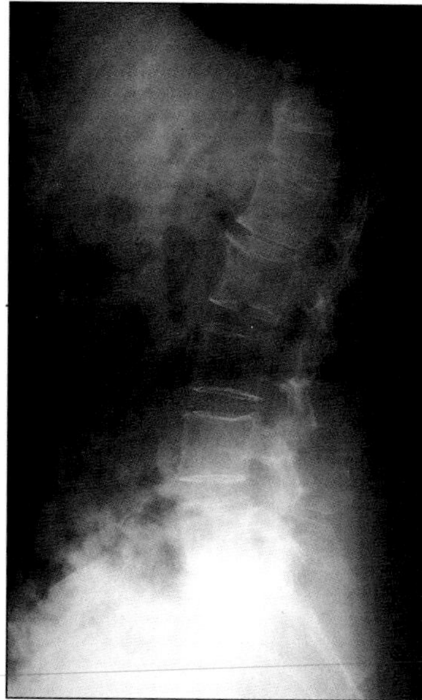

250 Picture framing and a compression fracture of the spine.

251

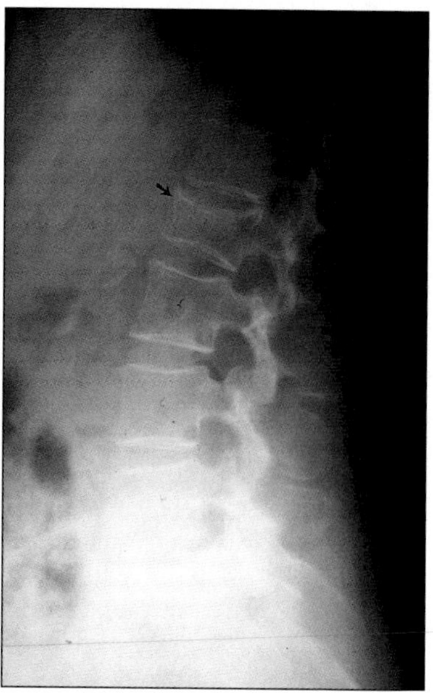

251 The arrow in this figure indicates 'fishmouthing' of L1; framing is also apparent.

252

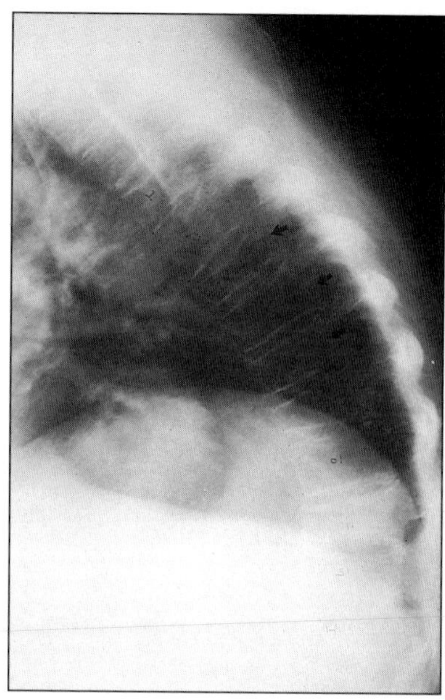

252 A wedge fracture of T7 and T8 and progressive loss of height in T6, T7 and T8. Loss of height in T9 and T11 less evident.

253

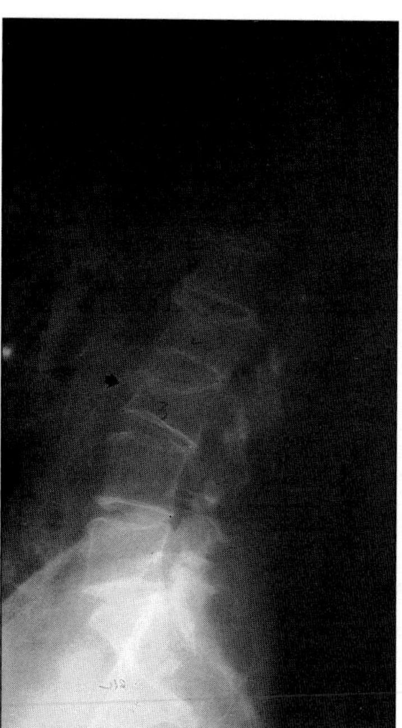

253 The arrow in this figure indicates anterior loss of height of T8.

254

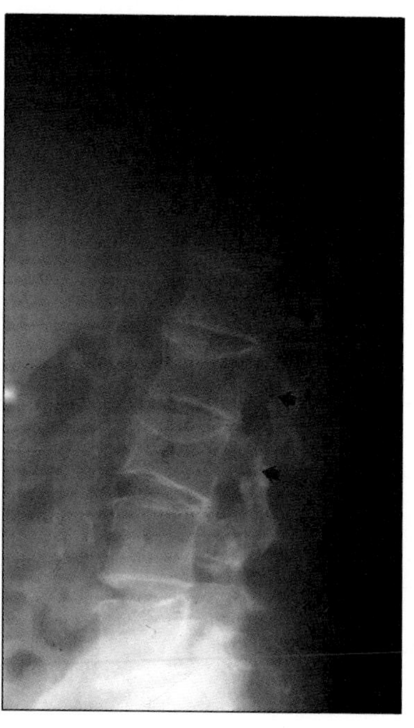

254 This is the same X-ray as **253** but the arrows indicate early and late progression of wedge fractures of L1, L2 and L3.

255

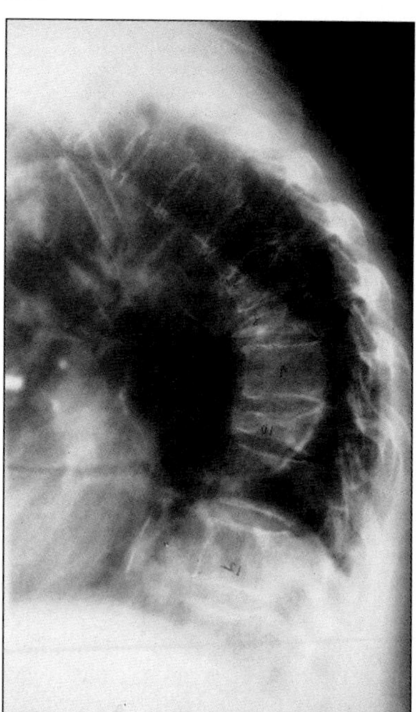

255 An X-ray showing a loss of anterior and posterior height.

256 A close-up of anterior loss of height in T11.

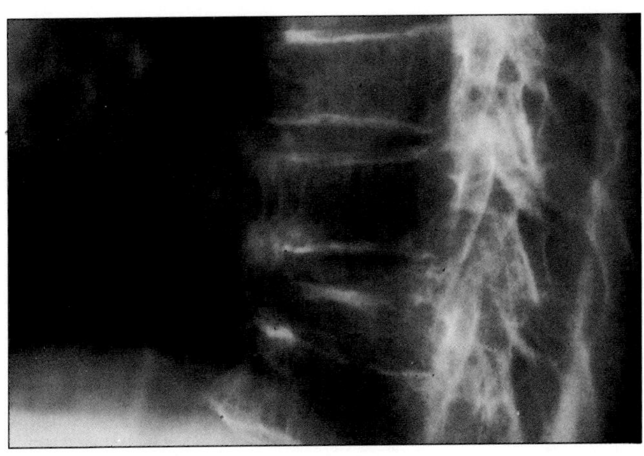

Apparent demineralization of bone may result from a haemangioma (**257, 258**). Wedge deformities may infrequently represent residual change from Scheuermann's disease or a previous traumatic fracture. Attempts have been made to classify the shape of vertebral anterior wedging; an angle ranging from 15–25% (lowering height anteriorly rather than posteriorly) has been proposed. Complete compression fractures cause a reduction of at least 25% in both anterior and posterior height compared to adjacent normal vertebrae. Graduated semi-quantitative grading scales have been developed to produce an overall spinal index (the sum of the grades from T4 to L5). The Mayo Clinic group and others have proposed elaborate scoring systems.

257 Demineralization of the bone as a result of a haemangioma.

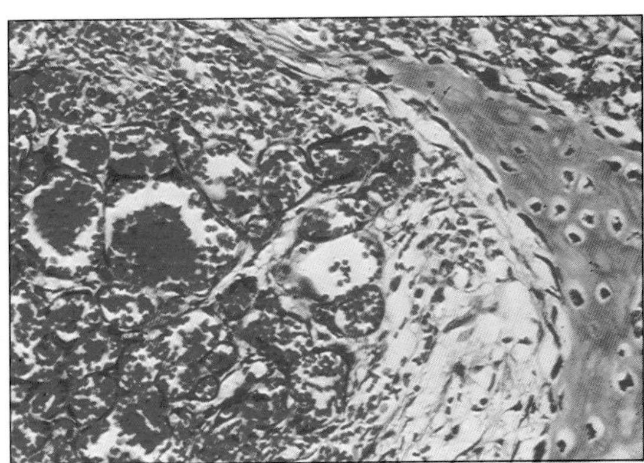

258 Haemangioma.

Bone loss in the appendicular skeleton is most apparent when there is a predominence of cancellous bone in the ends of the bones. The medullary canal is widened and the cortices of the long bones are thin. This picture is characteristic of Type II osteoporosis (**259**), whereas in Type I (or high turnover states) there is loss of both endosteal and intracortical bone.

The trabecular structure of the proximal femur has been studied in detail by Singh who has proposed the Singh index. As bone is lost, distinct areas of trabeculae are resorbed in a predictable order, based on the mechanical stress encountered by the trabeculae (**260, 261**). One difficulty with the Singh index is the high variability with different observers in clinical use.

259

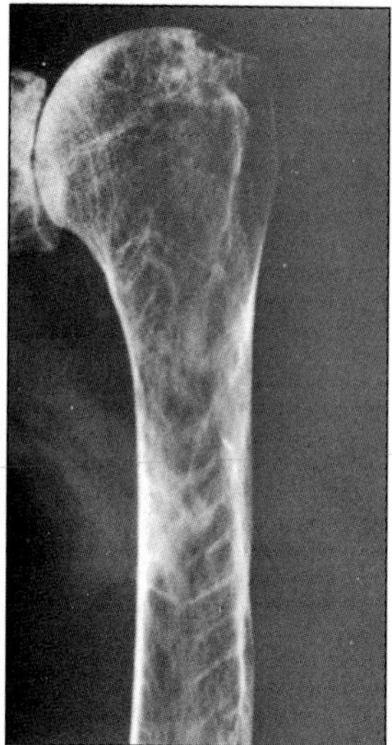

259 Type II osteoporosis is seen in a humerus with thin cortices and a widened medullary cavity.

260

261

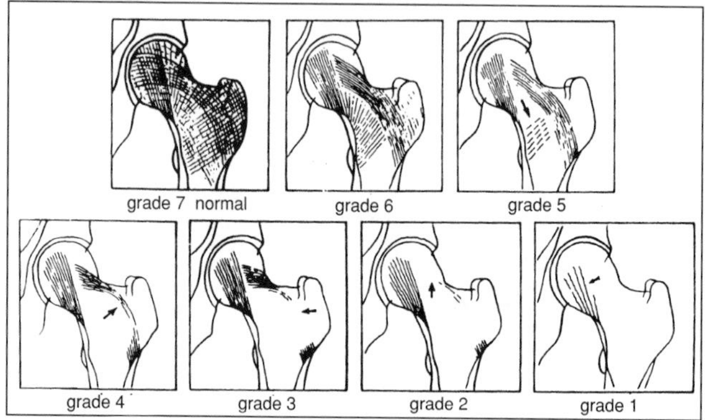

260, 261 Trabecular pattern in the Singh index.

262

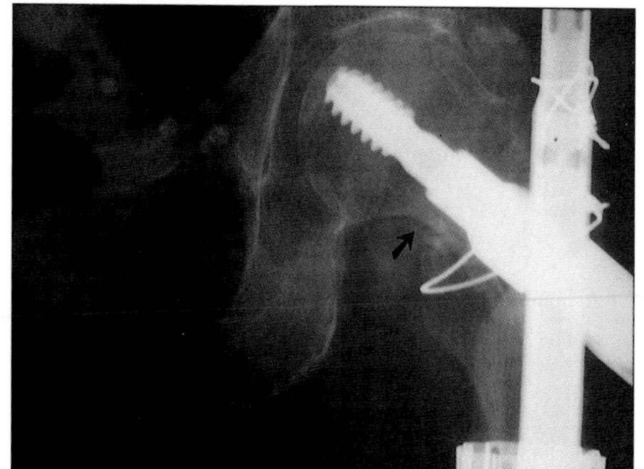

Fractures of the femur and some of the orthopedic fixation devices used in their treatment are shown in (**262–265**).

262 The arrow indicates an intramedullary rod in the left femur in a fracture which extends from the femoral head to the shaft.

263

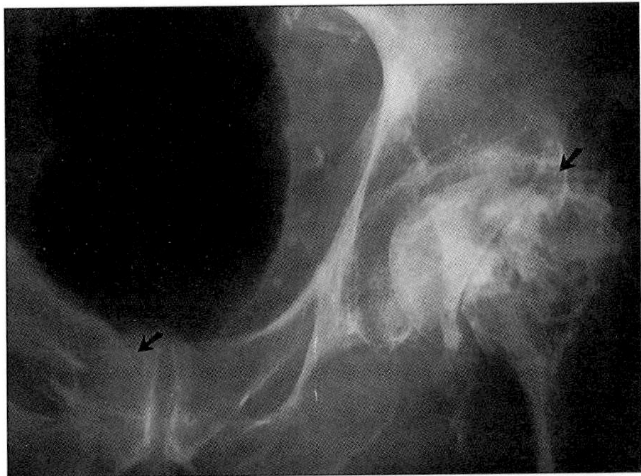

263 The arrows indicate a fracture of the left femoral neck and right superior pubic ramus.

264

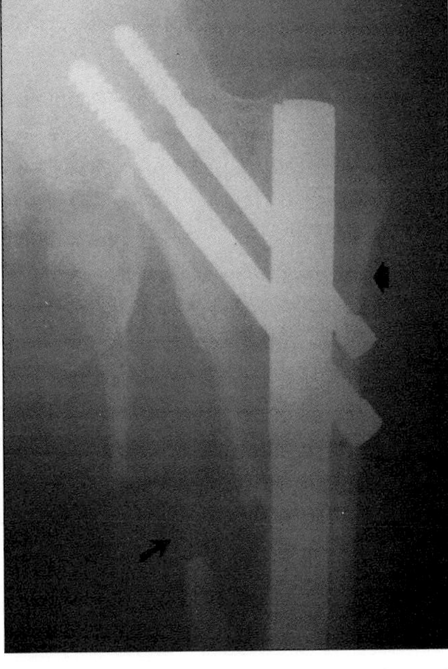

264 The arrows indicate a comminuted fracture of the left femur with an intramedullary rod.

265

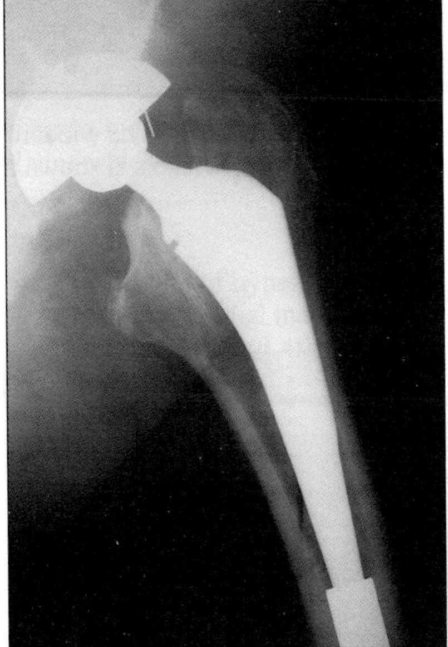

265 This X-ray shows a total hip replacement after the patient sustained a fracture of the left femur.

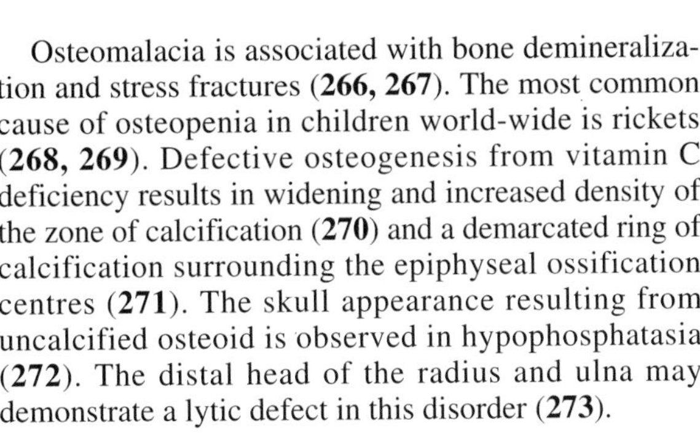

Osteomalacia is associated with bone demineralization and stress fractures (**266, 267**). The most common cause of osteopenia in children world-wide is rickets (**268, 269**). Defective osteogenesis from vitamin C deficiency results in widening and increased density of the zone of calcification (**270**) and a demarcated ring of calcification surrounding the epiphyseal ossification centres (**271**). The skull appearance resulting from uncalcified osteoid is observed in hypophosphatasia (**272**). The distal head of the radius and ulna may demonstrate a lytic defect in this disorder (**273**).

266

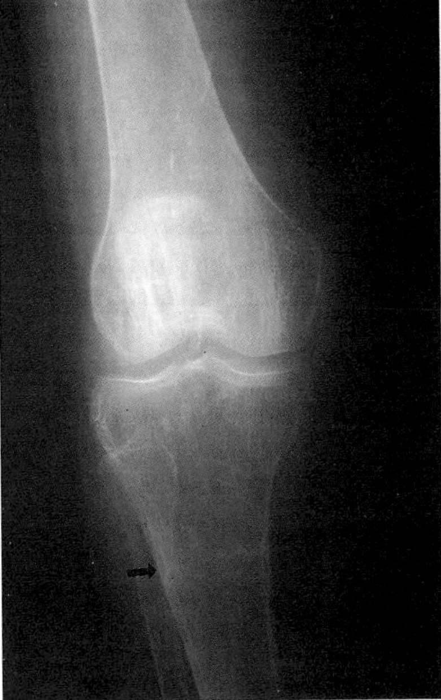

266 Osteomalacia; the arrows indicate stress fractures in proximal tibia.

screening is concerned. A task force of the American Osteoporosis Foundation recommended four conditions when bone mineral density should be evaluated:

- In oestrogen-deficient women, where the information will be used to decide on hormonal replacement therapy. Women who are 1 S.D. below the optimal value should receive hormonal replacement therapy or alternative anti-resorptive treatment. For those who have a value greater than 1 S.D. above the mean no further measurement is usually necessary, whereas those who are between ± 1 S.D. should have a repeat measurement taken in 3–5 years to determine if the risk has increased substantially as a result of rapid bone loss.
- In patients with vertebral abnormalities or roentgenographic osteopenia, bone mineral measurements should be used to confirm the presence of osteopenia. Roentgenographic diagnosis of osteopenia is grossly inaccurate; even the appearance of true fractures may not be indicative of osteopenia, and may only represent previous trauma, juvenile epiphysitis, positioning of the roentgenographic or normal variations in vertebral body shape.
- In patients receiving glucocorticoid therapy to diagnose low bone mass.
- In patients with asymptomatic primary hyperparathyroidism to identify those with severe skeletal disease. A Consensus Development Conference held in Denmark in 1990 recognizes another important clinical indication: the monitoring of treatment efficacy *(Table 24)*.

Other techniques that are not widely available or are still in the stage of development, include total body neutron activation analysis with whole body counting, Compton scattering, and research-oriented CT scans. The use of sonic waves has recently been introduced with the hope that this method may reflect bone fragility (in addition to bone density). An ultrasound instrument and a typical report are shown in **298** and **299**.

Table 24. Some potential indications for bone mass measurements.

Screening for fracture risk
- Unselective (mass screening)
- Selective
  - Patient concerns
  - Risk factors
- Before starting treatment for other reasons

Diagnosing osteoporosis in patients with vertebral abnormalities

Monitoring
- Non-responders to therapy
- Identifying 'fast losers'

Evaluating high-risk patients
- Amenorrhoea
- 1° or 2° hyperparathyroidism
- Steroid treatment
- Anticonvulsant therapy
- Thyroid replacement
- Anorexia nervosa
- Alcoholics
- Other diseases
- Multiple atraumatic fractures
- Disuse

298

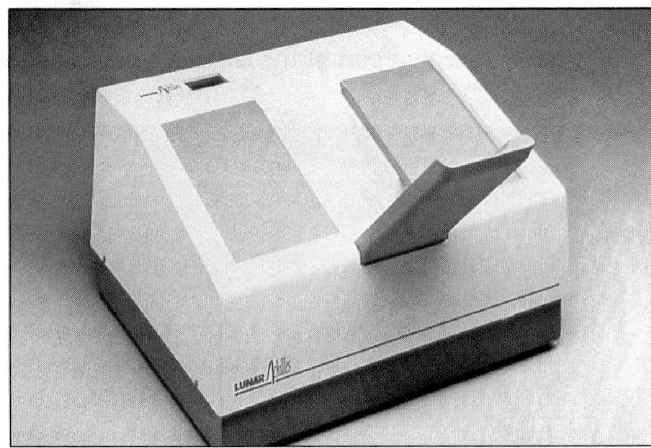

299

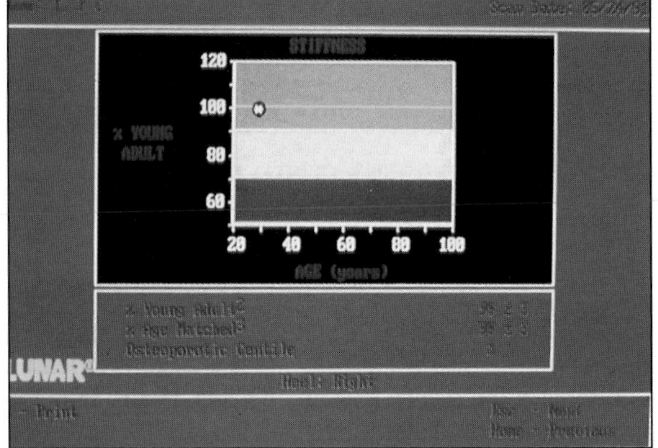

298, 299 An ultrasound instrument (**298**) and a report produced from it (**299**).

8. Treatment of osteoporosis

Introduction

Following a thorough clinical evaluation of the patient who has suffered an osteoporotic fracture, particularly of the spine or hip, the approach to treatment must be one of rehabilitation. In addition to increasing bone mass the goals include restoration of a positive outlook on life, increasing physical activity, restoration of independence, improvement of insomnia and anorexia through treatment of depression, pain relief, withdrawal from narcotics, restoration of muscle mass and strength, avoidance of fractures, and improvement in posture.

The acute phase – vertebral fracture

The back pain that results from a crush fracture in postmenopausal osteoporosis is sudden and severe. It may be confined to the vertebrae but may travel around the rib cage on one side or both into the front of the chest to the abdomen. Occasionally, the pain appears worse in the anterior aspect or even the flank. Osteoporotic fractures have been confused with heart attack, kidney stones, cholecystitis, pancreatitis, dissecting aneurysm, and herpes zoster. Tenderness in the spine is present on examination which leads to an X-ray and the discovery of a vertebral fracture. The history preceding the pain is useful in the diagnosis in that the patient very frequently has either fallen backwards or lifted a heavy object in the position of flexion of the spine. Often, the pain is not related to a preceding mechanical stress. As much as 2–20cm of height can be lost as a result of compression fractures. Kyphosis develops and the spine is shortened so that the arms are disproportionately longer than the trunk. The abdomen has less space for its intestinal contents and abdominal organs, and a potbelly or protuberant abdomen develops. The hips become flexed to maintain balance and many women walk with their feet spaced further apart and take slower steps. If this posture is allowed to persist, muscle atrophy ensues and chronic pain due to changes in configuration of the spine develops with the result that the patient is more likely to fall. Loss of confidence, fear of falling, and concern for loss of independence may all contribute to depression.

Severe pain persists for 3–6 weeks. During the first 3 weeks most patients remain in bed much of the time and are given narcotics to relieve the pain. Recently recommendations have been made to mobilize patients immediately using a brace. However, most patients, even if ambulatory during this time, will require significant bed rest. Patients are given stool softeners, and use a hard mattress with an egg crate. If the patient cannot find a comfortable position in bed it is recommended that she lies on her back with the knees flexed, with a thin pillow to support the head and regular size pillows placed below the knees to keep them flexed and another pillow between the legs. Massage may be used for pain relief, and heat can be applied through an infra-red lamp. Within 2–3 weeks non-narcotic analgesics may be substituted. It may be necessary for the patient to use a walker for ambulation at first (**300**). Activity is gradually increased to the pre-fracture level. Initial exercises should be mild, including walking or

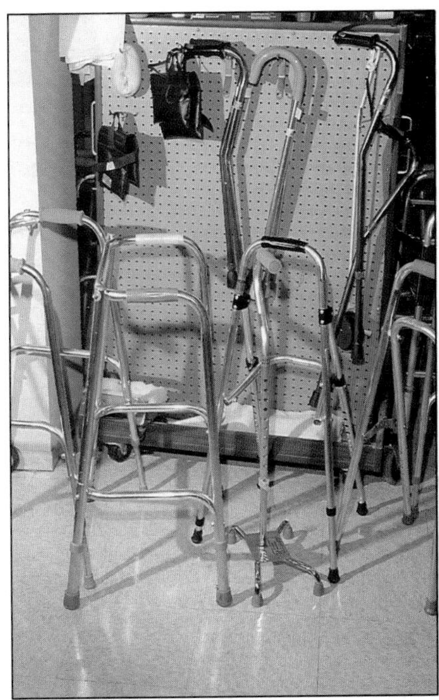

300

300 Assistive devices.

exercising in a heated pool. Pain medication can then be reduced or eliminated. Physical therapy is a mainstay of treatment in this early phase, following which patients should be enrolled in a physical therapy programme designed for treatment of osteoporosis.

Physical therapy in vertebral osteoporosis

In the patient with established osteoporosis an evaluation must be made of pain and its mechanism, mechanical dysfunction, muscle strength, gait, posture, balance, and depressive symptoms. Fear of injury must also be assessed. The goals of physical therapy are to correct mechanical dysfunction by reducing kyphosis, maintaining lordosis, aligning the hip, knee and foot, and providing external support if needed. An exercise programme should be taught in classes by physical therapists and patients should continue these exercises indefinitely at home. The objectives of exercise in women who have suffered a spinal fracture are different from those used in the prevention of osteoporosis. Their objectives are to strengthen the trunk and the muscles around the femur, to restore confidence, to maintain joint mobility, to improve co-ordination, to reduce pain by correcting mechanical imbalance, to improve posture, to increase muscle strength in the upper and lower extremities, to prevent bone loss from immobilization, and to practise relaxation techniques. Commonly used modalities include the use of ice, ultrasound, transcutaneous electroneuro stimulation, and myofascial release (**301**). Flexion exercises are avoided. Exercises to improve balance are prescribed. An education programme is essential in enabling the patient to understand the changes in body image, to reduce the fear of injury, or falling, and to increase compliance with a rehabilitative programme. In addition to the exercise program that will be described (much of which was developed at the University of Connecticut), the patient is encouraged to initiate a walking programme. The strenuous, bone-loading, osteogenic exercises prescribed for prevention of osteoporosis will result in fracture and should be avoided at this stage. However, it is important to realize that the patient with a vertebral fracture has as low a bone density of her femur as patients who have already had a hip fracture, and that an increase in the muscles of the hip, as well as improvement in balance are critical programme goals.

301

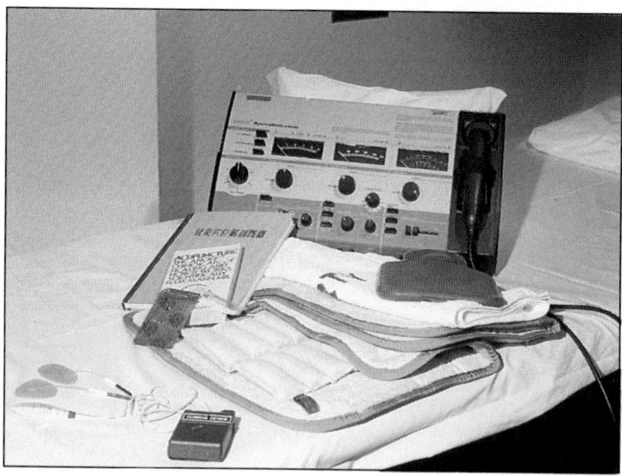

301 Non-narcotic pain relievers.

The use of orthoses remains controversial. In most instances the orthosis should be used only as a temporary device that can be discarded following a programme of physical therapy. Its primary use may be the provision of bracing during the acute fracture phase to permit ambulation. The purposes of spinal bracing are to decrease pain, protect against any further injury, and prevent or help correct a deformity that follows a vertebral fracture. Braces accomplish these goals by providing trunk support, limiting motion, and attempting to realign the vertebrae, but their effectiveness is usually limited. Lumbosacral supports are seen in **302–305**; the Taylor–Jewett brace is seen in **304**.

302

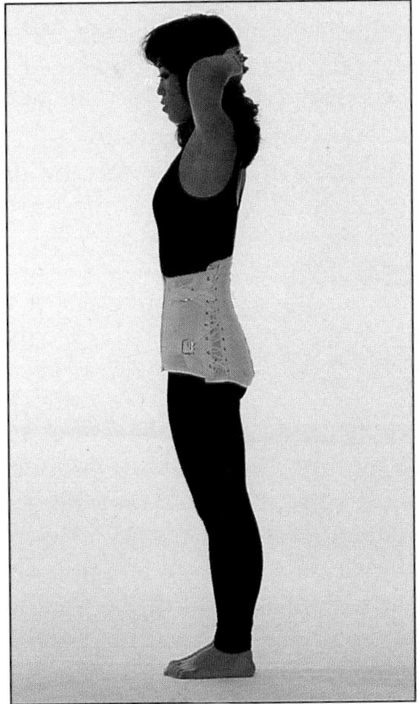

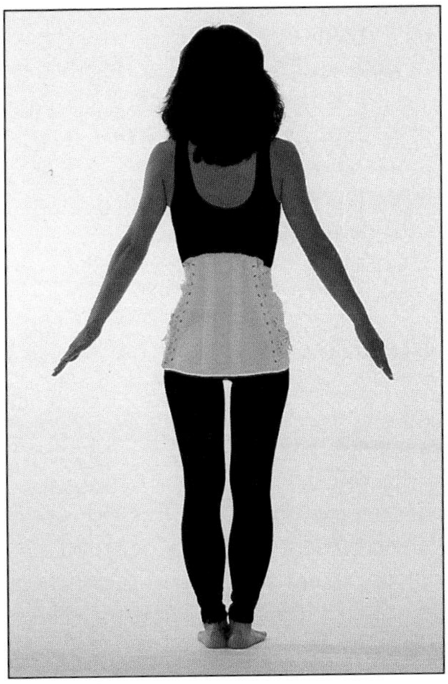

303

302–304 Lumbosacral supports.

304

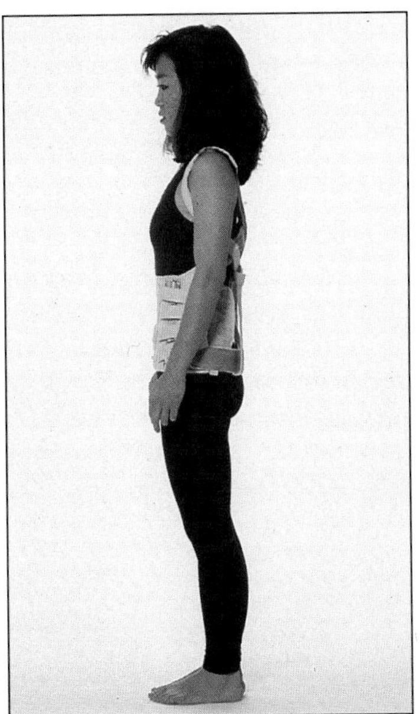

304 Lumbosacral supports *cont.*

305

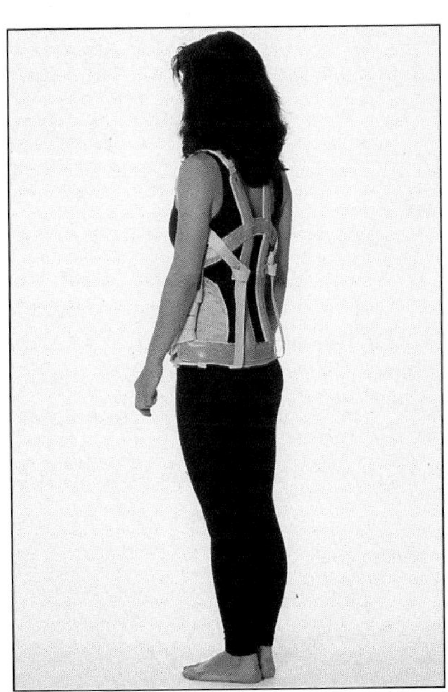

305 Taylor–Jewett brace.

The treatment of chronic pain

After several months following a vertebral fracture the patient should no longer have any pain. If it does persist the physician must re-investigate and ask the following questions:

- Was the diagnosis of primary osteoporosis incorrect? That is, does the patient have a malignancy or multiple myeloma?
- Are there any new fractures?
- Is the pain from pull on ligaments or from muscle spasm?
- Is an exercise programme causing the pain?
- Are microfractures occurring?
- Is the patient dependent on narcotics or depressed?
- How well does the patient tolerate pain?
- Is there secondary gain as a result of disability?
- Are the lower ribs rubbing against the pelvic brim, thus causing pain?

For the most part pain may be alleviated by the use of non-narcotic analgesics with physical therapy. Electrical stimulation may be tried as may other pain alleviation techniques, such as acupuncture, hypnosis, biofeedback and behaviour modification. Pain reduction may result from the use of small doses of an anti-depressant. It is important to be cautious with medications as some may increase the propensity to fall. A variety of over-the-counter medications may be used with massage to reduce muscle spasm. If these efforts are unsuccessful, then the patient should be referred to a pain clinic.

Fractures of the proximal femur

Although there are elaborate classifications of femoral fractures, for most purposes they can be considered as either fractures of the femoral neck or of the intertrochanteric region of the proximal femur. It is important to differentiate between these fractures because of the blood supply to the proximal femur which may be compromised in femoral neck fractures, resulting in loss of blood flow to the femoral head. Decisions concerning treatment of femoral neck fractures are made based on the degree of displacement of the fracture and the obliquity of the fracture line. The greater the displacement, the greater will be the disruption of the blood supply. Fractures with minimal displacement are often fixed in position with screws, pins, or plates. With more severe displacement the risk of avascular necrosis or of non-union is greater. In younger patients efforts are made to preserve the femoral head using fixation and bone-grafting. The results, in terms of the complications of avascular necrosis and non-union, are still far from ideal. Replacement of the femoral head with artificial devices may be required and is preferable in older patients. This procedure allows early ambulation and consequently earlier discharge from hospital. Densitometry has recently been used to assess the bone surrounding an implant.

Since intertrochanteric fractures do not compromise the blood supply to the femoral head, they are usually treated by internal fixation using rods, screws or plates.

Wrist fractures

The most common wrist fracture is the Colles' fracture. This fracture may extend into the joint, be associated with an injury to the distal ulnar, and can result in angulation and shortening of the wrist as well as dorsal displacement. Treatment is usually by manipulation and casting. In severely comminuted fractures, external fixation with pins in the bones on each side of the fracture may be required. It is important to realize that Colles' fractures are osteoporotic and that a patient who has fallen may have fractures of the humeral head as well as the neck of the humerus. In addition, a minimally displaced femoral neck fracture can be present. Thus, it is important to evaluate someone who has fallen for these other fractures as well.

Pelvic fractures

Non-traumatic fractures in the osteoporotic patient normally occur in the anterior aspect of the pelvis. They are usually confined to the ischium or pubis and are often unilateral, but may also involve bilateral fracture of the superior and inferior pubic rami. This area is not important in weight bearing and the fractures are stable. The patient remains in bed until he or she can tolerate ambulation. A walker is used for several weeks in the early stages of ambulation.

Treatment to increase bone density

An ideal drug for the treatment of osteoporosis is not yet available. Optimal characteristics of the medication would include the following: the drug should be safe; it should increase bone mass to a level such that there is no further risk of fracture (above the 'fracture threshold'); the new bone formed should be architecturally sound (i.e. it should be normal bone in composition and structure); the abnormal architecture that resulted from osteoporosis (loss of trabeculae) should be restored; and the medication should be easy to take and readily accepted by patients. Nonetheless, there are a variety of medications available that reduce bone loss and it is a realistic hope that there will be new ones which safely increase bone mass. The variety of drug mechanisms are indicated in *Table 25*.

Table 25. Classification of treatment mechanisms.

Inhibitors (reduce remodelling)
- Calcium
- Oestrogen
- Progesterone
- Testosterone
- Anabolic steroids
- Bisphosphonates

Activators (stimulate remodelling)
- Fluoride
- Growth hormone
- IGF-1
- Phosphates
- Low-dose parathyroid hormone

Stimulate calcium absorption
- Vitamin D and its analogues

Use of more than one drug (combination)
- Increase bone formation and decrease bone remodelling by simultaneous use of activators and inhibitors.

Sequential therapy
- Use of activator, then inhibitor, followed by a period of no drug treatment (rest) and then repetition of the sequence.

Inhibitors

Oestrogen

Hormonal replacement therapy is preferred for prophylaxis or treatment during the perimenopausal and early postmenopausal years. Nonetheless, oestrogen is effective in decreasing bone loss in the elderly as well; however, there is not yet a great deal of information concerning complications of hormonal replacement therapy in the frail elderly. Following initiation of oestrogen therapy the serum oestradiol level should be ascertained. A level of 50pg/ml or more is considered in the therapeutic range. Many physicians will add a progestogen for 14 days to the oestrogen regimen to minimize the risk of endometrial cancer. A variety of hormonal replacement regimens are under active investigation. Hormonal replacement therapy remains the treatment of choice for prevention of postmenopausal osteoporosis, and is generally prescribed for treatment in women who are within 10–15 years of the menopause.

Calcium

As stated earlier, an adequate calcium intake is important in all stages of life. Calcium requirement is greater in childhood, adolescence, pregnancy, lactation and old age. Therefore, it is recommended that elderly individuals with osteoporosis take between 1,500–2,000mg of calcium per day. This intake in the elderly will most likely only be accomplished by taking calcium supplements (see Chapter 4). In the elderly it is more likely that there is reduced gastric acid secretion which could result in decreased absorption of carbonate salts. As a result, if calcium carbonate is used, it should be given with meals when there is likely to be gastric acid secreted. Whenever there is a suspicion of reduced gastric acid, then it would be preferable to treat the patient with calcium citrate or calcium citrate malate. Since urinary calcium is highest in the evening, at least a portion of calcium citrate or citrate malate may be given at bedtime. For prophylaxis, those patients on a calcium-deficient diet will benefit most. An adequate calcium intake is provided with every other treatment regimen to ensure sufficient calcium for bone formation and to reduce the likelihood of secondary hyperparathyroidism. In the homebound elderly, or individuals in a nursing home, it is wise to supplement the diet with vitamin D, although some nursing homes have used ultra-violet light exposure. Supplements can be given in the amounts of 400–800IU per day. There is no evidence that megadoses of vitamin D are useful in the treatment of primary osteoporosis and they may even be harmful.

Calcitonin

Calcitonin (**306**) is an alternative therapy in the prevention of postmenopausal bone loss in women who cannot or will not take oestrogens. Calcitonin, in the treatment of established osteoporosis, does not have the risks associated with hormonal replacement therapy. Consequently, it is preferred for older women. Therapeutic regimens include medication given by injections, suppository, or nasal spray. Calcitonin injections are usually given at bedtime. Injectable calcitonin (salmon and human) produces side effects of flushing, nausea, vomiting, diarrhoea, abdominal cramps, and urinary frequency in as many as 30% of patients. However, these symptoms are not enough to produce discontinuation of the drug in all but a small percentage of patients. These symptoms are obviated by the use of the intranasal spray. The intranasal administration of calcitonin has been shown to be effective in the prevention of postmenopausal bone loss in European studies. **307** shows a reduction in fracture rate in patients treated with calcitonin and calcium, which should always be included with antiresorptive therapy. There is some evidence for an analgesic effect of calcitonin which may be greater with intranasal administration.

306

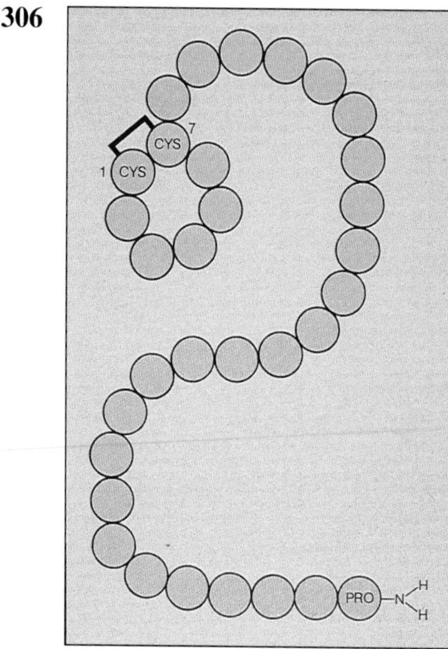

306 The structure of calcitonin.

307

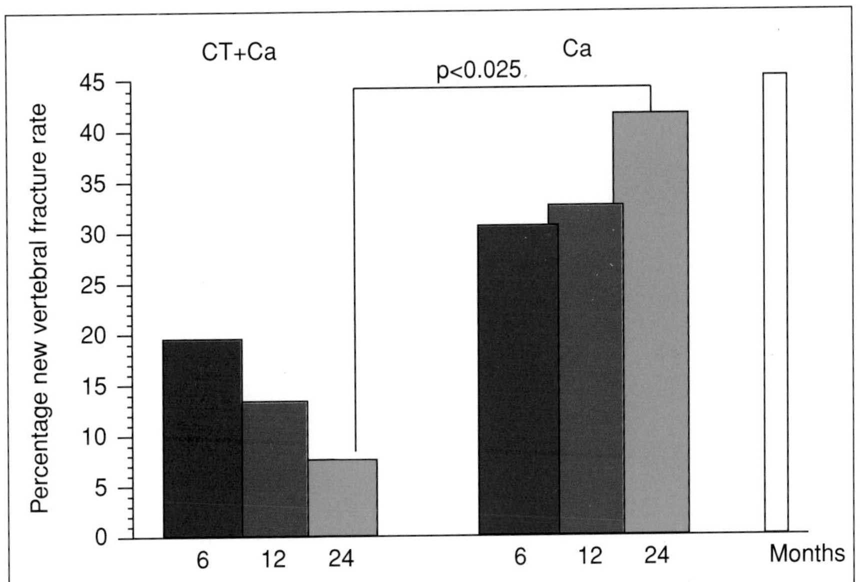

307 Bar chart showing the reduction in fracture rate in patients treated with calcitonin and calcium.

Bisphosphonates

The bisphosphonates are analogue compounds of pyrophosphate. There are second and third generations of these drugs and etidronate, clodronate, elendronate, tiludronate, and pamidronate have all been investigated for use in osteoporosis. These agents decrease bone resorption by chemisorption onto bone crystal. Two recent studies have demonstrated an improvement in spinal bone mass. Some studies suggest that they are successful in preventing postmenopausal bone loss. The bisphosphonates, with the possible exception of pamidronate, appear to have minimal side effects. However, it is not yet clear which therapeutic regimens are optimal and for how long these medications should be given. Their very long half-life in bone raises concerns about inhibition of microfracture repair. Thus, with these agents, it will be important to demonstrate that the quality of bone is normal and that they result in a reduction in fracture rate. **308** shows the fracture reduction rate with the cyclic use of etidronate.

308

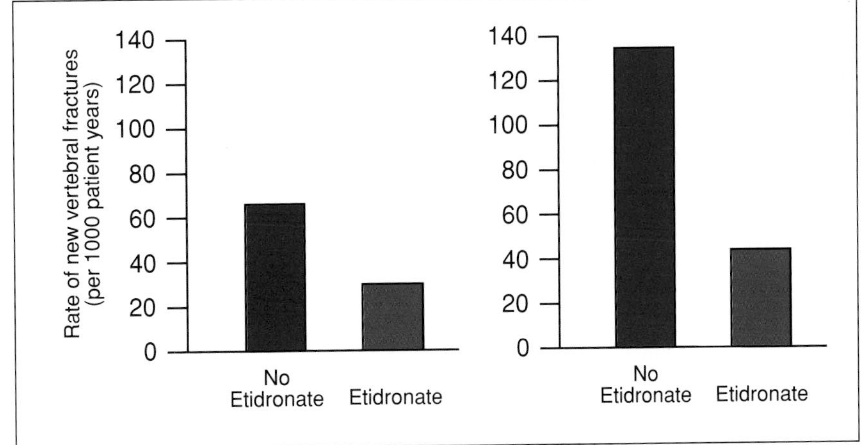

308 The fracture reduction rate with the cyclic use of etidronate.

Thiazide diuretics

Thiazide diuretics increase urinary calcium retention. There is sufficient epidemiological evidence that thiazide diuretics may prevent osteoporotic fractures. Clinical trials are currently being planned or conducted.

Tamoxifen

Although tamoxifen has not been studied as a primary therapy for osteoporosis its effect on bone appears to be that of inhibition of bone resorption. This agent will have wide-spread use in women with breast cancer and may have beneficial effects in preventing bone loss. Consideration is being given to the use of tamoxifen in the prevention of breast cancer and osteoporosis.

Activators

Sodium fluoride

Sodium fluoride administration in pharmacologic doses increases bone density of the spine and trabecular bone volume in the iliac crest bone biopsies. Early histomorphometric studies demonstrated a mineralization defect following fluoride use. Seventy per cent of patients appear to respond to the therapy and patients have been classified as 'responders' and 'non-responders'. The smallest dose for which an increase in bone mass has been demonstrated is 30mg per day and the bone response appears to be dose-dependent. Fluoride has a direct effect on osteoblastic function. Although fluoride has been available for many years, most reports concerning its use have been in uncontrolled series. Two large controlled clinical trials using 70mg sodium fluoride failed to demonstrate a statistically significant benefit when it was used to reduce vertebral fractures and, at the same time, they showed an increase in appendicular fractures. The use of fluoride is a good example of an agent which increases bone density, yet the quality of the bone formed is poor. However, although the bone formed is of poor quality, it is hoped that the increase in bone mass might be sufficient to reduce fracture rate. Proponents of fluoride therapy believe that there is a narrow therapeutic window and that doses up to 50mg a day of sodium fluoride may have a beneficial effect. Moreover, the appendicular fractures were related to high serum levels of fluoride. New formulations developed using fluoride salts have reduced some of the gastrointestinal effects experienced with this medication. Sodium fluoride therapy should still be considered experimental.

Anabolic steroids

There is some evidence that anabolic steroids increase bone formation, whereas other studies suggest that their primary effect is similar to oestrogen and that they reduce bone resorption. Long-term use may produce virilization and adverse effects on carbohydrate and lipid metabolism, and on liver function.

Parathyroid hormone

Daily subcutaneous injections of low doses of a synthetic aminoterminal fragment of human parathyroid hormone has been shown to increase trabecular bone density of osteoporotic men and women, on bone biopsy. Since the physiologic effect of parathyroid hormone is anabolic on bone, the rationale for this therapy is reasonable. However, studies undertaken with parathyroid hormone and parathyroid hormone combined with calcitriol have shown positive effects only for a limited period of time. It is likely that this agent will prove to be of benefit only in combination with other medications and its use remains experimental.

Growth hormone

Growth hormone clearly produces an increase in the activation of bone remodelling; acromegaly is associated with an increase in bone mass. Initial studies with growth hormone given alone, however, have failed to demonstrate an increase in bone density. The use of physiologic replacement therapy with growth hormone in elderly individuals to restore IGF-1 levels to young adult levels, has resulted in the maintenance of bone density. The use of other growth factors, such as IGF-1 and TGF-β, in the treatment of osteoporosis remains to be investigated. Such agents hold the greatest promise for future regimens that increase bone mass.

Calcium absorption stimulants

Calcitriol and other vitamin D metabolites

Since osteoblasts contain receptors for calcitriol, it has been hoped that vitamin D analogues might not only reduce bone resorption through an increase in calcium absorption but also stimulate bone formation. The difficulty with the use of these drugs has been that, in order to obtain high serum levels to stimulate osteoblastic activity, they must first pass through the intestine which results in hypercalciuria. The vitamin D analogues do increase bone density. The use of high doses of 1,25-dihydroxyvitamin D or 1,α–hydroxyvitamin D may be associated with significant side effects in occasional patients. However, in a study of 13,000 patients in Japan, hypercalcaemia occurred when a dose of 0.25μg BID of 1,α–hydroxyvitamin D_3 was used in only 0.4% of patients.

1,α–hydroxyvitamin D_3 is used widely in Japan where it has been shown to be useful in prophylaxis as well as in the treatment of established osteoporosis and the reduction of fracture rate. A study undertaken in New Zealand involving 622 patients also showed a low incidence of hypercalcaemia when a lower dose was used, and a reduction in fracture rate (**309**). The therapeutic window remains narrow with the available vitamin D analogues, and calcium supplements should not be used with them. Urinary and serum calcium must be followed in these patients. Vitamin D analogues under development may avert the first pass intestinal effect and may increase bone formation.

309

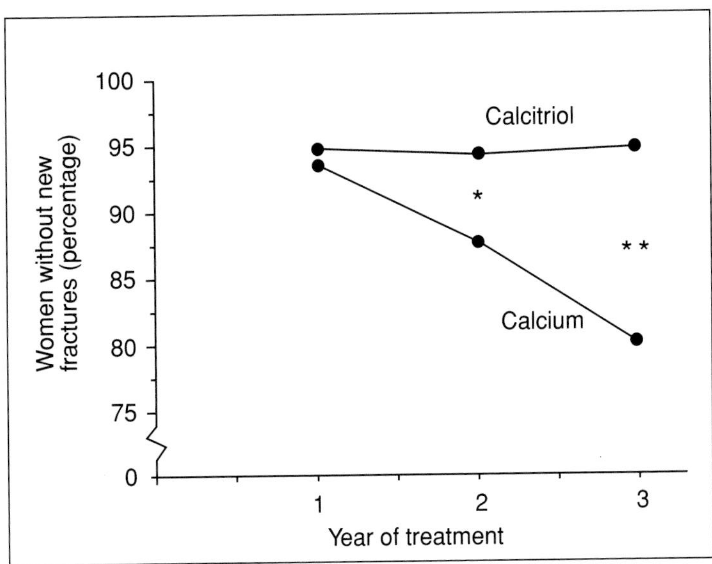

309 Graph showing a reduction in fracture rate with a vitamin D analogue (∗, $p<0.05$; and ∗∗, $p<0.01$).

Combination drug therapy

In this regimen an agent that reduces bone resorption is given simultaneously with one that increases bone formation. Calcium supplements are taken as they are with other treatment regimens. A variety of combination therapies have been studied. However, there have been no large scale clinical trials that would lead to the definitive recommendation of these treatment regimens.

Sequential therapy

Sequential therapy is also known as ADFR (activate, depress, free, repeat) and utilizes the knowledge of bone remodelling dynamics to attempt to increase bone mass. Remodelling sites are activated throughout the skeleton in an attempt to produce both an increase in bone remodelling units and skeletal coherence. Activators of bone remodelling such as parathyroid hormone, growth hormone and oral phosphates have been used. Following activation, the bone resorption is depressed by an inhibitor of bone resorption such as calcitonin or a bisphosphonate. Theoretically, the resorption phase does not continue to completion whereas the signal for bone formation has been initiated. Thus, during the free phase there is no treatment so the remodelling sequence is allowed to continue into the formation phase. It is believed that the new bone formed will be in an amount equivalent to that which would have been resorbed if an inhibitor of bone resorption had not been given. After a cycle is completed the sequence is repeated over and over again (**310, 311**). ADFR therapy remains experimental and no clinical trials have appeared which clearly demonstrate its efficacy. The timing and dosage of agents remain under investigation.

310

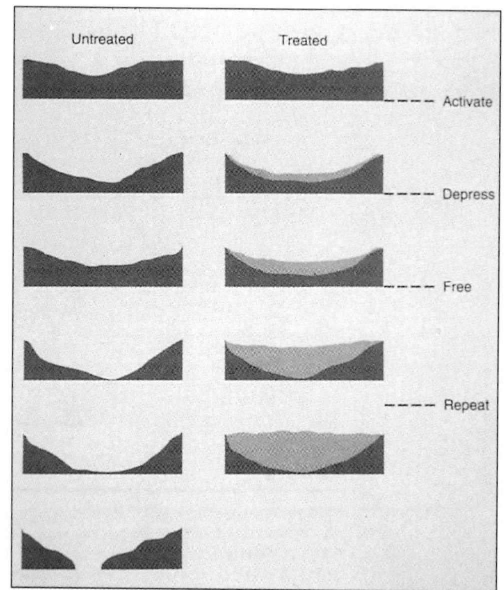

310 The theoretical changes in bone remodelling balance in ADFR therapy.

311

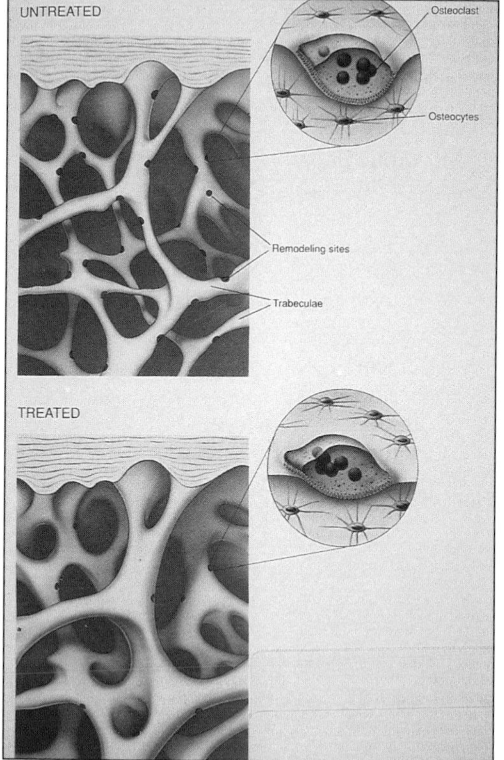

311 Before and after treatment with an ADFR regimen. The trabeculae are thickened, and active resorptive sites are reduced.

Secondary osteoporosis

Management of some of the secondary osteoporoses may be mentioned under drug therapy. Few controlled trials to support current practices have been undertaken. For prophylaxis of glucocorticoid induced osteoporosis the following have been recommended:

- Maintain the lowest glucocorticoid dose, eliminate other causes of osteopenia, increase calcium intake to 1500mg per day, reduce hypercalciuria with a thiazide, provide up to 800IU of vitamin D per day.
- Increase vitamin D intake to produce the suppression of PTH with the avoidance of hypercalciuria (maintain urine calcium at 2.5–3.5mg/kg body weight). If osteopenia occurs (or is present), the addition of an antiresorptive medication may be tried, e.g. gonadal steroids, anabolic steroids when appropriate, or calcitonin or a bisphosphonate.

For prophylaxis of anticonvulsant osteopenia, adequate calcium and vitamin D should be added with a programme of exercise; again, larger doses of vitamin D (or 25-hydroxyvitamin D) are indicated if bone loss ensues or osteopenia is present.

Exercise programme for the individual with established osteoporosis

The risk of injury from exercise in the elderly is much greater than in young people and the benefits in terms of prevention of bone loss are also less in those who already have osteopenia. Special problems such as emphysema and coronary artery disease or Parkinson's disease may be present. Moreover, problems to be addressed include postural changes and disorders of body mechanics, gait disturbances, muscle contracture, and joint inflexibility. Spinal flexion exercises have been shown to increase the incidence of vertebral fractures in women with osteoporosis. Increasing bone mass through a weight-lifting programme is clearly out of the question for most osteoporotic patients, although it is important to appreciate that women with vertebral osteoporosis have severe femoral osteopenia and that improvement in lower extremity strength (and muscle mass) is an important therapeutic goal for all osteoporotic patients.

The objectives for osteoporotic individuals to be aimed for by exercising include: restoration of confidence; improvement in joint mobility; improvement in posture; an increase in muscle mass and strength; reduction of pain; reduction of stress; improvement in cardiorespiratory fitness; and prevention of bone loss. A good way of beginning exercise after a fracture is through a walking programme or swimming in a heated pool which improves mobility and increases confidence. Useful exercises include: back extensions, postural stretching, deep breathing, abdominal muscle strengthening, exercises that increase strength in the lumbar extension and gluteus maximus, increase the musculature of the hip, and exercises that improve posture and co-ordination while reducing stress.

Flexibility is the ability of a joint to move through its full range of motion. Static flexibility is a measure of the total range of motion at a joint, whereas dynamic flexibility is a measure of the resistance to movement. To maintain proper alignment of the spine in an osteoporotic patient, the abdominal and hamstring muscles must be strengthened and the erector spinal and hip flexors must be stretched. For osteoporotic women both static stretching and proprioceptive neuromuscular facilitation stretching should be used. Exercises should be supervised at first, and then incorporated into a home programme. The theraband is a useful device. Many of the exercises illustrated below were developed at The Osteoporosis Centre of the University of Connecticut.

The T'ai Chi walk should begin and end the workout. Follow with stretching exercises (**312**), and those included in the prevention programme, including stand tall, wall glide, heel raises, shoulder and leg, front leg and side stretch. Back extension, back tighteners and the lower back stretch are practised as well. The additional recommended exercises are shown in **313–334**.

312

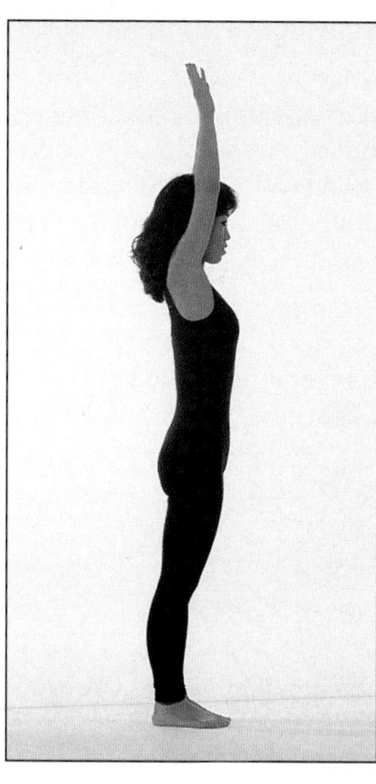

312 Stretching exercises.

313

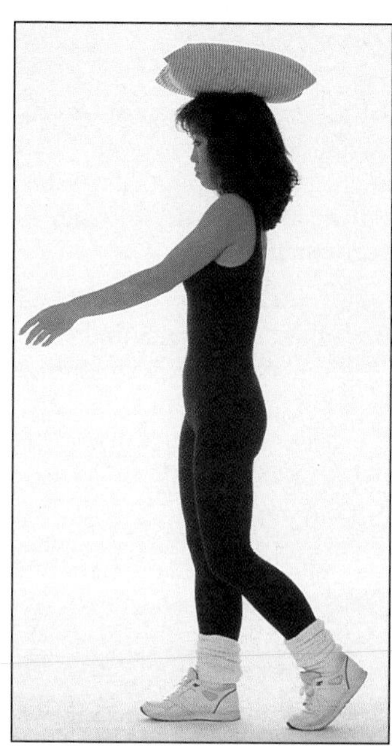

313 Erect walking. Walk with your chin in, head held high, shoulder blades slightly pinched, and stomach flat. Land lightly on your heels. Make sure your knee is lined up over your second toe at all times. Practise with a small, firm pillow on your head.

314

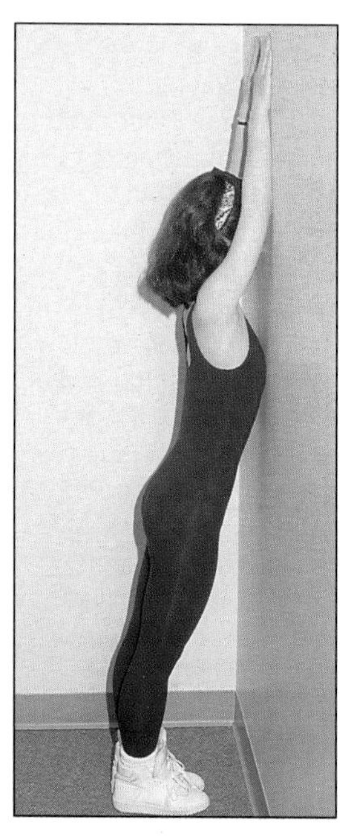

314 Wall arch. Facing a wall, stretch your arms up while taking a deep breath in. Concentrate on flattening your upper back as you flatten your stomach. Reach up with one arm while stretching down with the other.

315

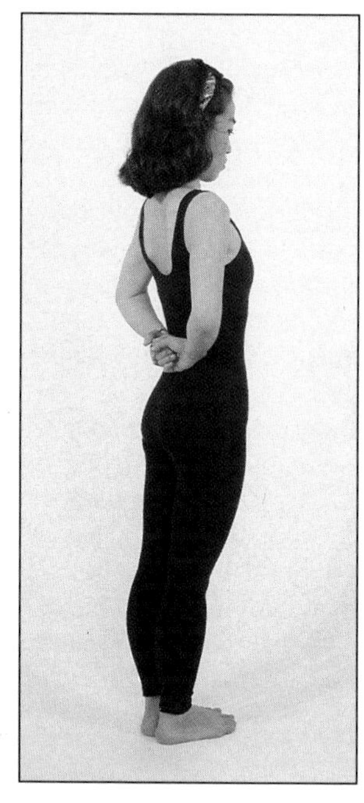

315 Standing back bend. Put your two fists on your lower back. Arch backwards slowly, while taking a deep breath. Repeat, this time placing the fists on the middle back. Repeat again with fists on the upper back. Keep your stomach muscles contracted during each stretch.

316

316 Wall standing and pelvic tilt. Place your feet 30cm away from a wall. With bent knees, have your head, shoulders and upper back touching the wall. Use a towel roll at the level of your waist to support your lower back. Slide up and down, bending the knees and keeping the back flat. As the back and stomach muscles improve, the feet can be placed closer to the wall while keeping your stomach muscles contracted. Hold the 'wall sits' for up to 30 seconds, 4 times per day.

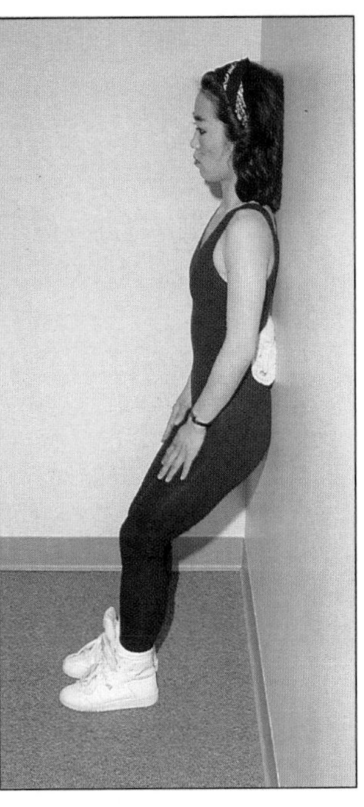

317

317 Chin pulls. Pull your chin in as if you could move it to the back of your neck. Look straight forward, not up or down. Keep your head high. Push down on your knees to help your back become as erect as possible.

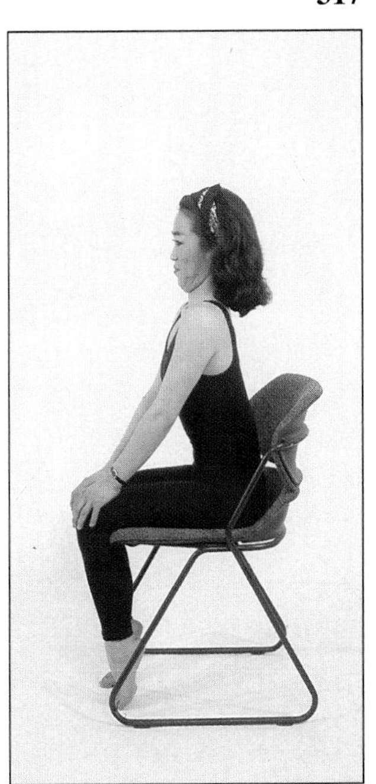

318

318 Isometric posture correction. Stand as tall as you can with your chin in, not up. Place your palms against the back of your head. Push against your scalp while simultaneously pinching your shoulder blades together and tightening your stomach. Build up a 'resistance' to the count of three. After holding for 3 seconds, slowly release over 3 more seconds. Maintain an erect posture throughout this exercise.

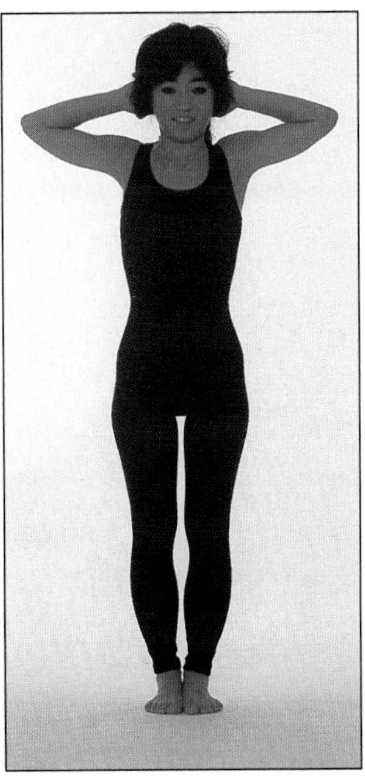

319

319 Chair rises. Sit on the near edge of a chair and repeatedly rise to a standing position. Keep your knees and feet hip-width apart at all times. Lean forward slightly as though you feel weight on your toes as you stand and sit. This exercise is best done in two or three sets during the day. A set is equal to 5–20 chair rises, as tolerated.

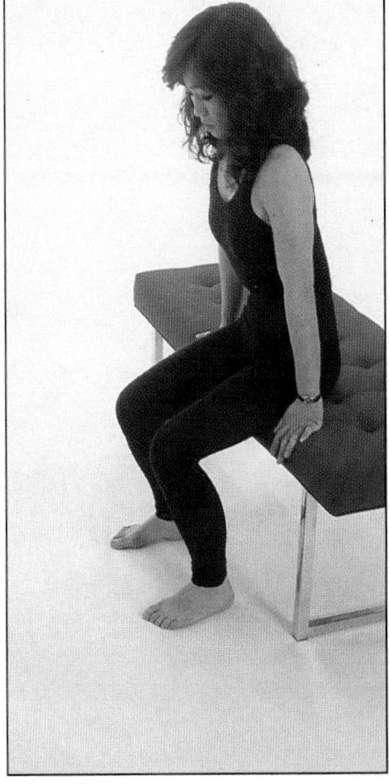

320

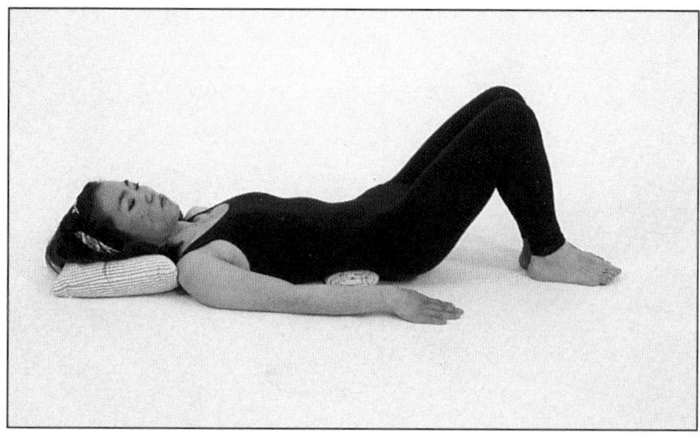

321

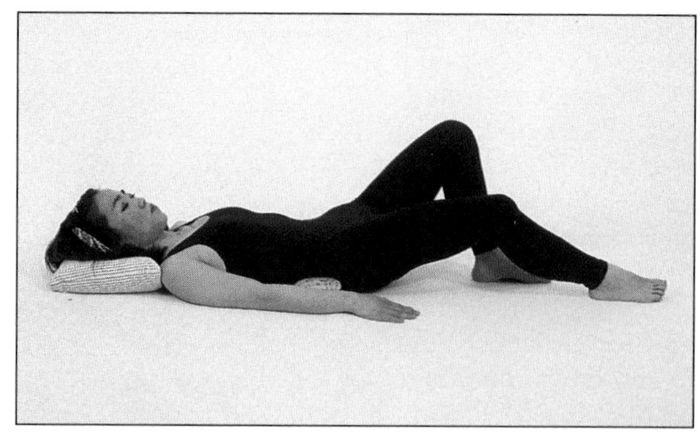

320, 321 The bridge. Lie on your back, keeping your knees bent. Press your head and shoulders down. Lift trunk, hips, and thighs. Relax, repeat. Eventually do with one leg only (alternating left and right leg).

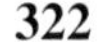

322

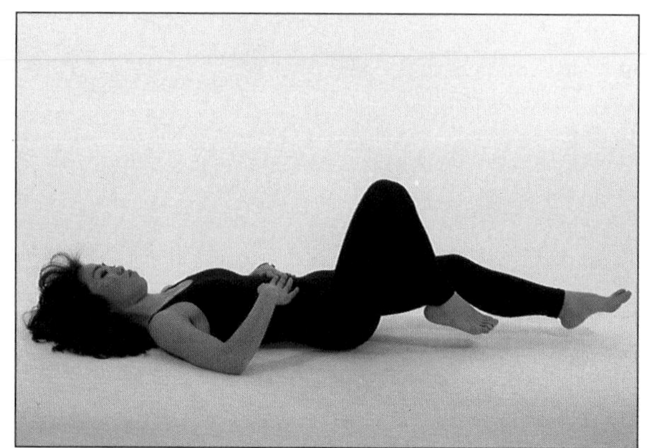

322 Pelvic tilt with leg slide. Lie on your back with knees bent. Press your back onto the mat, pulling your lower abdominal muscles down and in as if to tuck your stomach under your ribs. Your buttocks will lift slightly (not your whole back). Use a towel roll under your back for comfort if necessary. Slide one leg as far as you can, maintaining the tilt. Return to original position, relaxing the tilt. Repeat with the other leg.

323

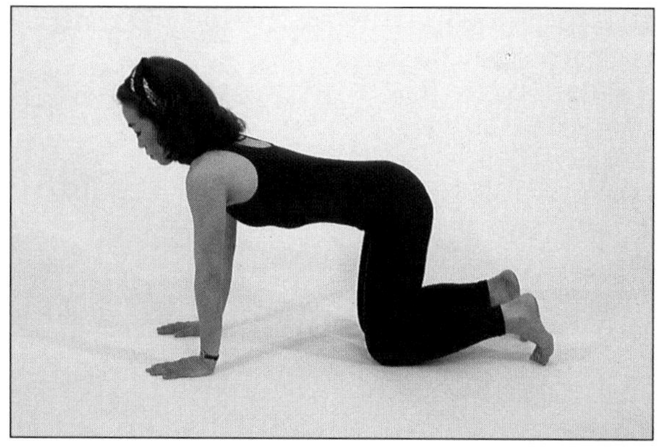

324

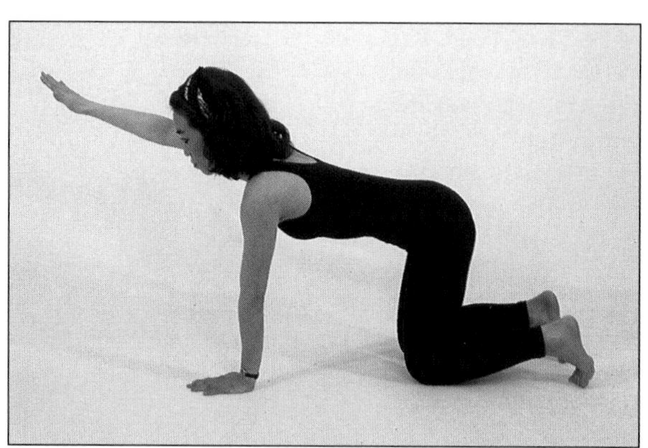

323–326 All fours arm/leg lifts. Get on your hands and knees (**323**). Hands should be directly under the shoulders; knees should be directly under hips. Your back should be flat or slightly arched. The stomach should be held flat. Alternate lifting each arm, holding for 3 seconds (**324**).

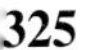

325

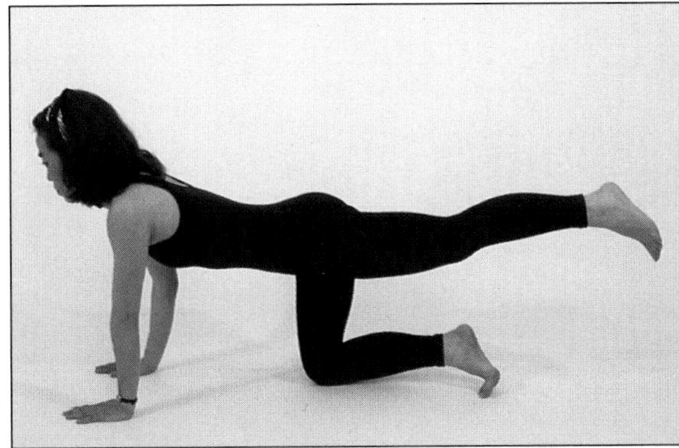

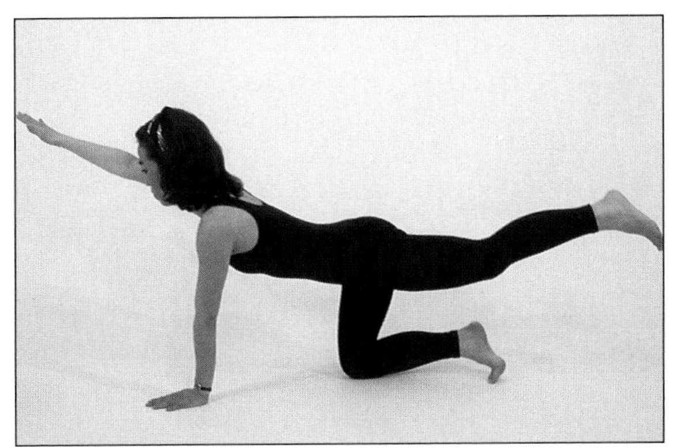

326

323–326 cont. Alternate lifting each leg, holding for 3 seconds (**325**). After you can do this comfortably, lift your right arm and left leg simultaneously (**326**). Then alternate: lift left arm, right leg. Follow with the cat stretch (see **333** and **334**).

327

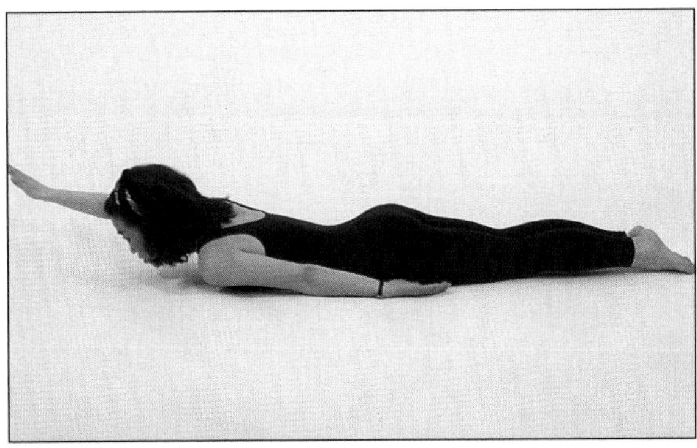

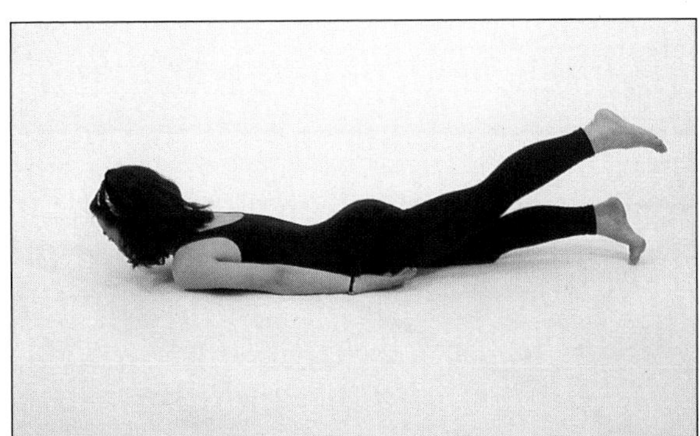

328

327–329 Prone arm/leg lifts. Lift one arm from the shoulder and hold for 3 seconds. Relax. Repeat with the other arm. Then, lift one leg from the hip and hold for 3 seconds. Relax. Repeat with the other leg. Lift the right arm and the left leg simultaneously and hold for 3 seconds. Relax. Repeat with the opposite arm and leg. Follow with the cat stretch.

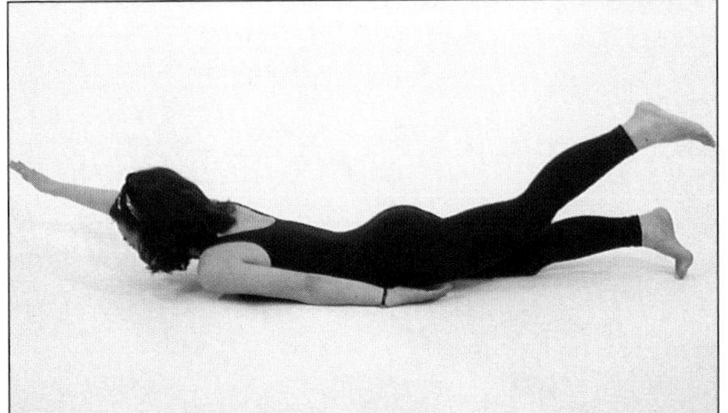

329

330

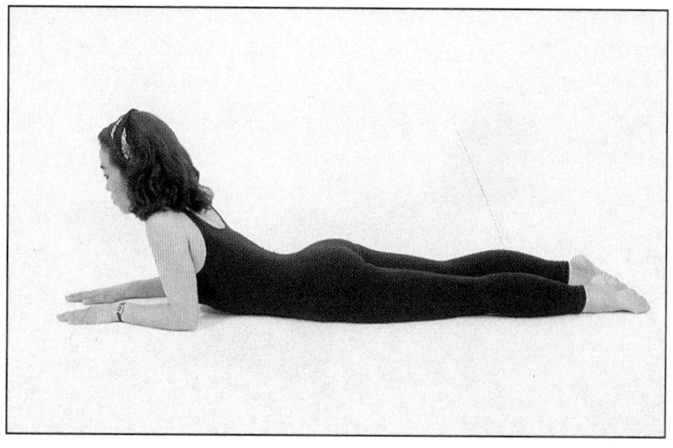

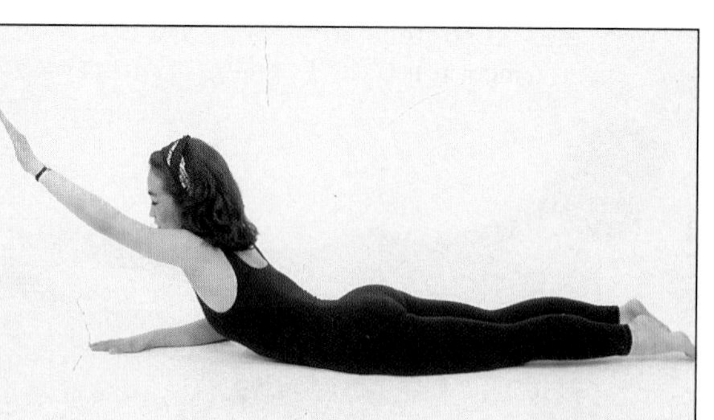

33

330–331 The elbow prop. As an alternative to sitting or lying on your back, try this position with or without a pillow. Attempt to stay in this position for 30 minutes per day—starting at 5 minutes initially—while watching television or reading. By passively decompressing the vertebrae and discs, this position helps reverse damage caused by poor posture. A good back exercise in this position is to reach each arm forward, alternating left and right arms. Follow with the cat stretch.

332

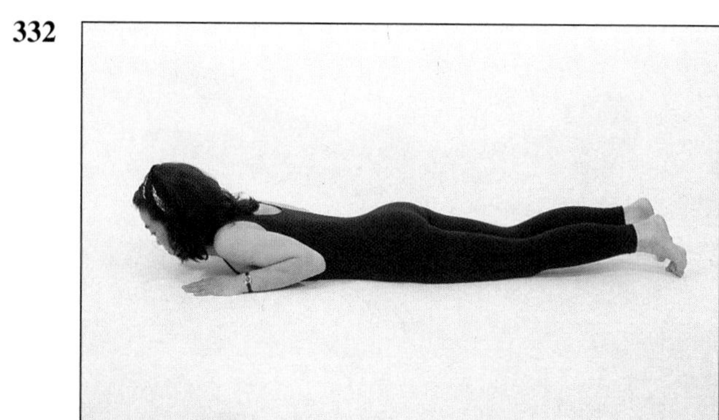

332 Prone press-ups with deep breathing. Start out in a conventional 'push up' position. Arch your back pinching your shoulder blades together. As you rise up, inhale; as you go down, exhale. Keep elbows partially bent to protect the back. Use a pillow under your stomach for comfort, if necessary. Make sure you don't lift your pelvis. Follow with the cat stretch.

333

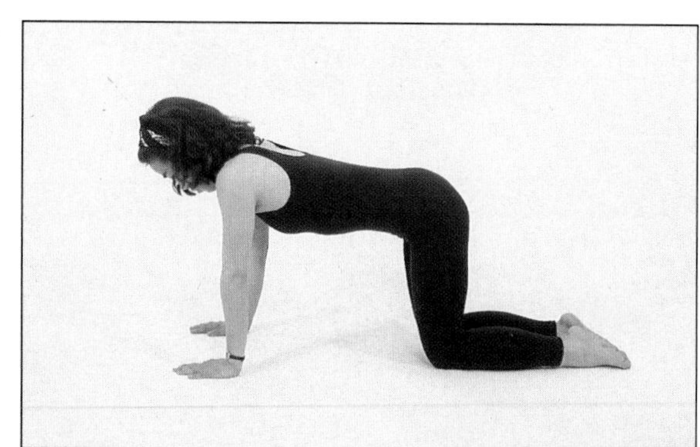

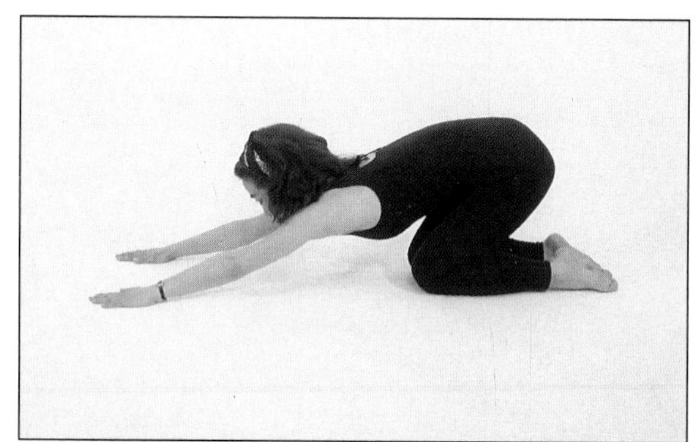

334

333, 334 The cat stretch. Get into the all-fours position, then sit back slightly and stretch out your arms in front of you as far as possible. Exhale as your stretch and relax.

Theraband (a stretchable plastic) can be used to provide resistance. It is used to stretch the arms (**335**), 'marching' in a chair (**336**), and in bending and straightening the knees. Exercises can be performed with the use of a theraband on a locked door, standing or sitting (**337–341**). More recommended exercises are shown in **342–344**.

335

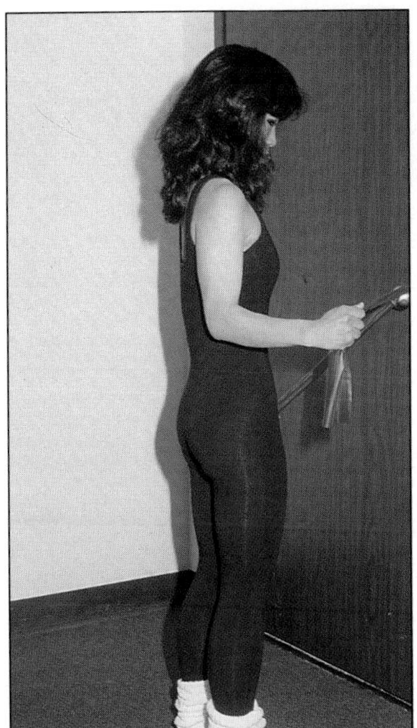

336

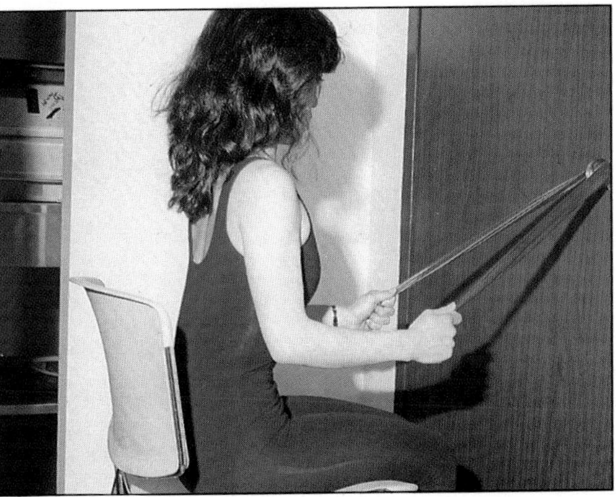

335, 336 Arm-stretching exercises using a theraband.

337

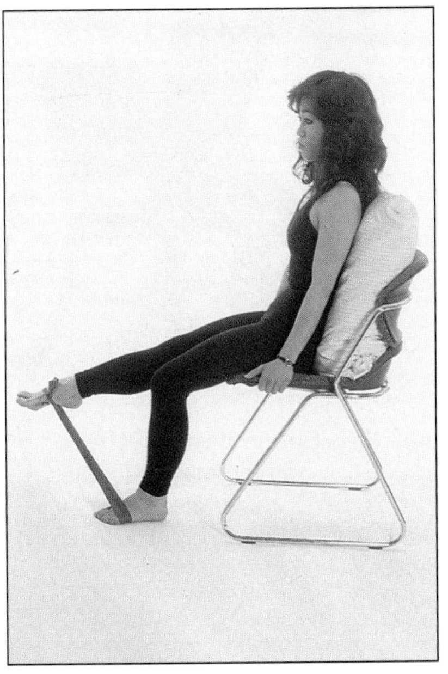

338

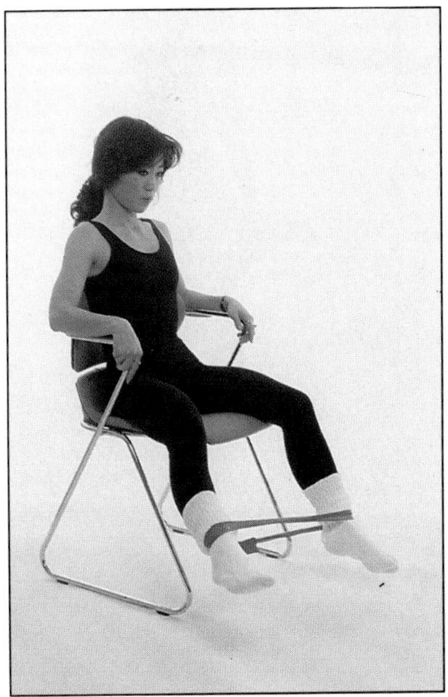

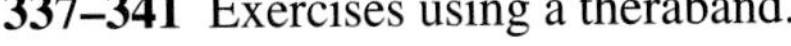

337–341 Exercises using a theraband.

339

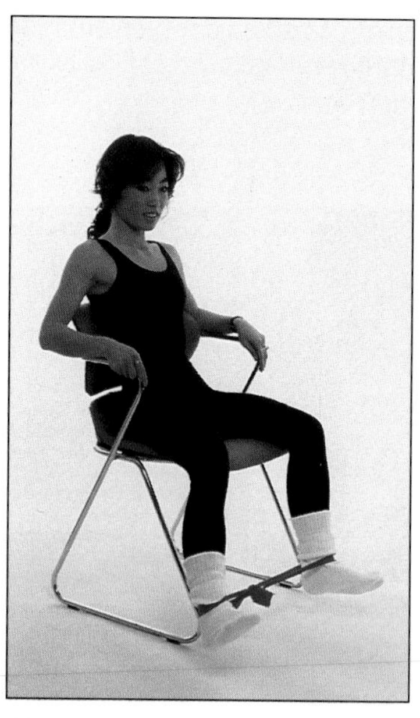

340

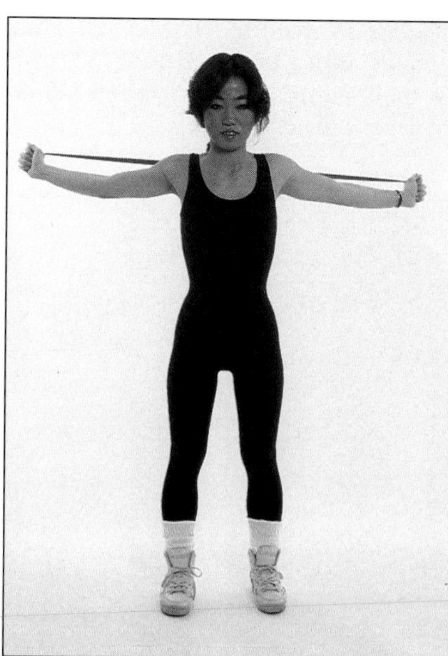

341

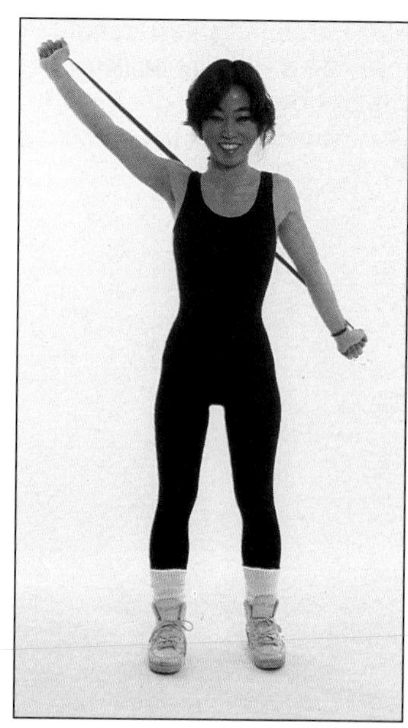

337–341 cont. More exercises using the theraband.

342

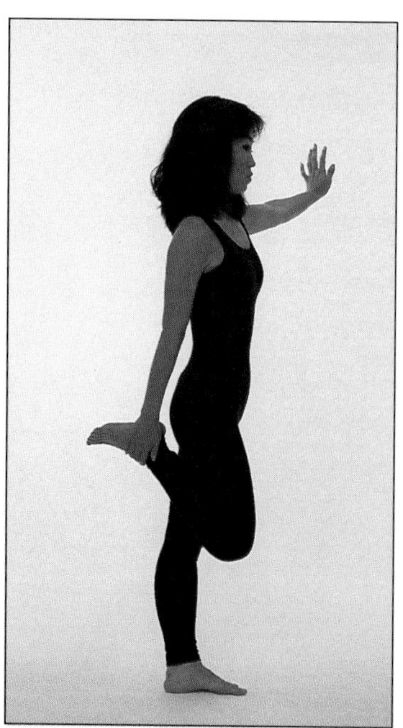

342 Position control. Stand with the fingers supporting first one leg and then the other. Repeat on each leg for 10 counts, then repeat on each leg for 20 counts.

343

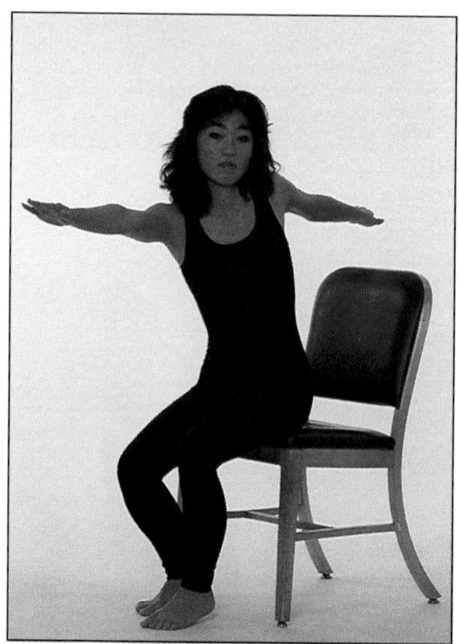

343 Position control. Sitting on a chair, turn and look to the left and to the right. Repeat with your arms stretched sideways. Perform each 10 times.

350

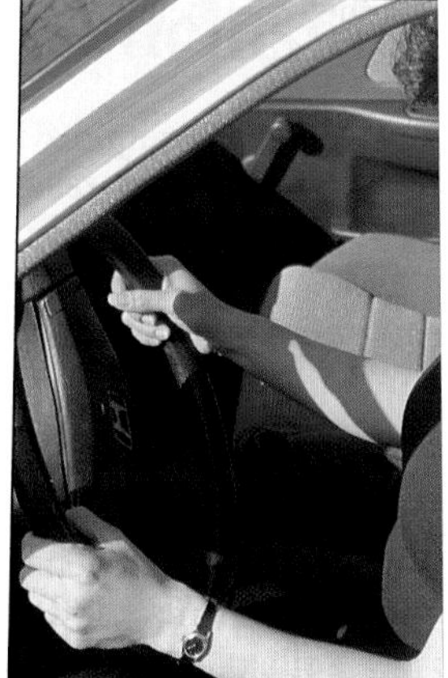

350, 351 Correct (**350**) an

352 Corr
out of a c

353

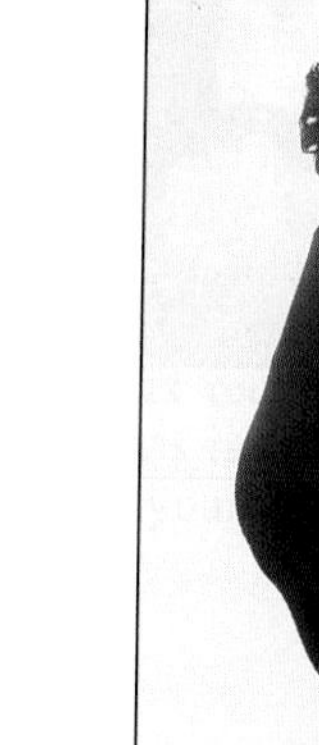

353, 354 (

344 Position control. Stand and slowly pick up an object from a table. Place it on a chair and then back on the table. Repeat 10 times.

344

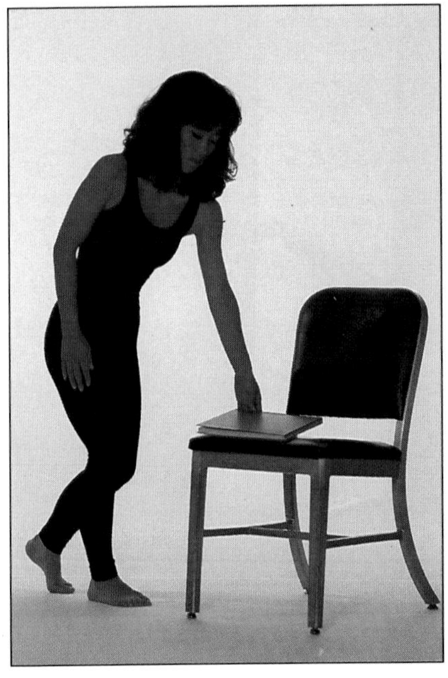

Exercise must also be incorporated into the daily routine of osteoporotic patients. There must be constant awareness of posture. In order to strengthen the lower extremities, it is valuable to do chair rises about 20 times, 3 times a day. The wall slide should be done mid-day with an ultimate goal of 20 times daily. It is also worthwhile to climb stairs during the day, practising good posture, using a railing for assistance. Proper hip/knee and foot alignment should be practised. The toes are kept straight ahead with the knees rotated outward, lined up over the second toe. A walking programme is prescribed.

Postural 'Do's and Don'ts' (appropriate body mechanics) must be learned by women with spinal osteoporosis to promote good posture. The upper back is almost flat, the shoulders are pinched together, the abdomen is flat and the lumbar spine is arched backwards. In **345** and **346**, the correct and incorrect mechanics are shown for vacuuming, raking or sweeping. The knees are bent and movement forward and backward, and side to side (**345**) is encouraged rather than slouching and bending and twisting (**346**). Similarly, when brushing the teeth the knees are bent rather than bending over (**347**).

345

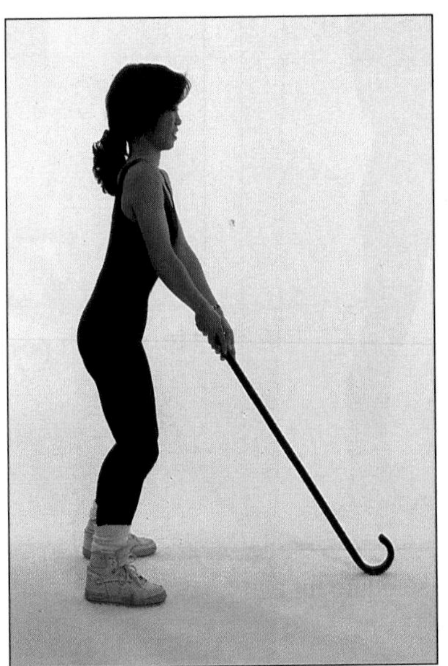

346

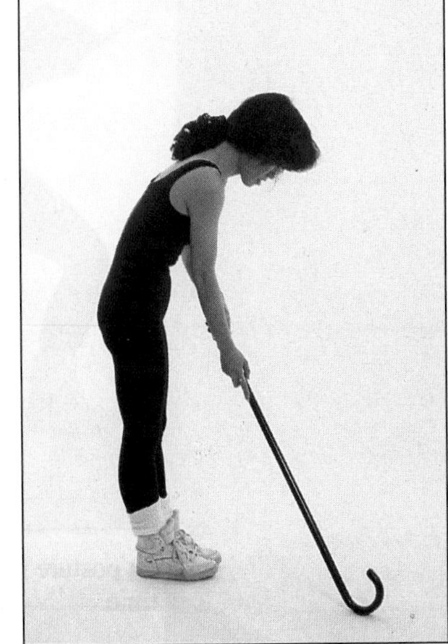

345, 346 Correct (**345**) and incorrect (**346**) postures for vacuuming, raking etc.

347

When standing for a
be placed on a stool a
(**348**). When sitting at
should be used behind
the chair should be adj
bend over, or a proppe
who sit at a job shoul

348

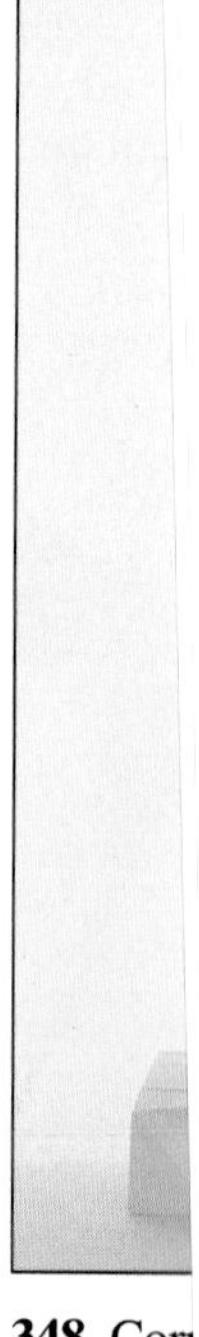

348 Cor
length of